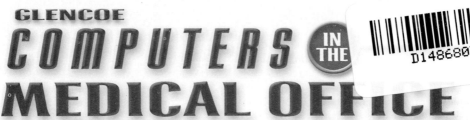

GLENCOE
COMPUTERS IN THE
MEDICAL OFFICE

3rd Edition

Includes MediSoft Advanced Data Disk

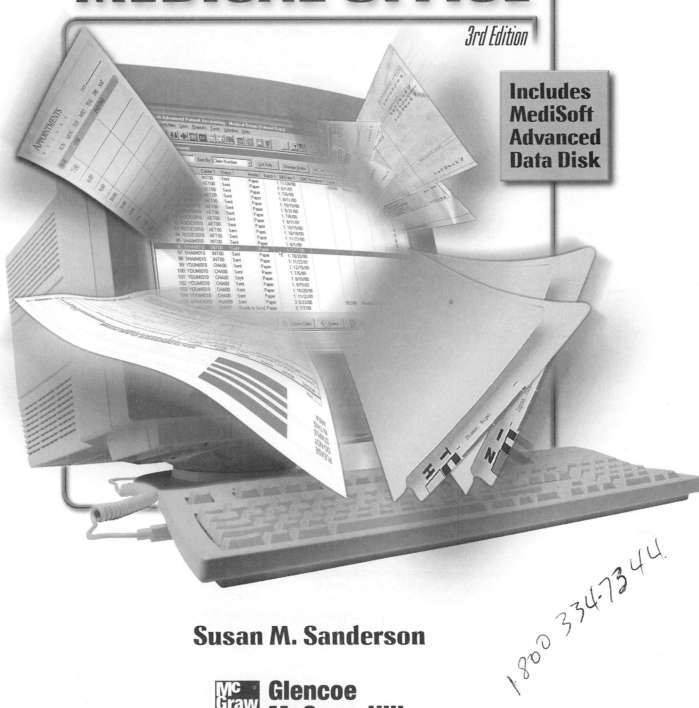

Susan M. Sanderson

Glencoe
McGraw-Hill

New York, New York   Columbus, Ohio   Woodland Hills, California   Peoria, Illinois

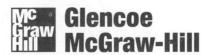

Library of Congress Cataloging-in-Publication Data

Sanderson, Susan M.
　　Computers in the medical office : using MediSoft for Windows : with student data disk /
　Susan M. Sanderson.—3rd. ed.
　　　p.　cm.
　　Previous ed. published under title: Glencoe computers in the medical office.
　　Includes index.
　　ISBN 0-07-823134-5 (pbk.)
　　　1. Medical offices—Automation. I. Sanderson, Susan M. Glencoe computers in the
　medical office. II. Title.
　R864.S26 2001
　651'.961' 0285—dc21

　　　　　　　　　　　　　　　　　　　　　　　　　　00-052536

Glencoe/McGraw-Hill

*A Division of The **McGraw·Hill** Companies*

Glencoe Computers in the Medical Office

Send all inquiries to:
Glencoe/McGraw-Hill
8787 Orion Place
Columbus, OH 43240-4027

ISBN 0-07-823134-5

　3 4 5 6 7 8 9 079 02

Codeveloped by
Glencoe/McGraw-Hill
and Chestnut Hill Enterprises, Inc.
Woodbury, CT

The Student Data Disk, illustrations, instructions, and exercises in *Computers in the Medical Office*
are compatible with the MediSoft Advanced Patient Accounting for Windows software available
at the time of publication. Adaptations may be necessary for use with subsequent versions of
the software. Text changes will be made in reprints when possible.

All brand or product names are trademarks or registered trademarks of their respective
companies.

CPT five-digit codes, nomenclature, and other data are copyright ©1999 American Medical
Association. All rights reserved. No fee schedules, basic unit, relative values or related listings
are included in CPT. Chestnut Hill Enterprises, Inc., and the AMA assume no liability for the
data contained herein.

All names, situations, and anecdotes are fictitious. They do not represent any
person, event, or medical record.

Contents

Preface

Demand for health care services is increasing, due to technological advances and to an aging population. Administrative duties in medical offices are also becoming more involved with technology. Computers are now used in almost all medical practices. Students who aim to find an administrative job in the health care industry will find that computer skills are often a prerequisite for employment.

This text/workbook, *Glencoe Computers in the Medical Office*, prepares students for administrative tasks in health care practices. The text/workbook introduces and simulates situations using MediSoft Advanced Patient Accounting for Windows, a widely used medical administrative software. While progressing through MediSoft's menus and windows, students learn to input patient information, schedule appointments, and handle billing. In addition, they produce various lists and reports, and learn to handle insurance claims both electronically and on paper. These invaluable skills are important in effective financial management of health care practices.

Although this text/workbook features MediSoft Advanced Patient Accounting for Windows, its concepts are general enough to cover most administrative software intended for health care providers. Students who complete *Glencoe Computers in the Medical Office* should be able to use other medical administrative software with a minimum of training.

TEXT/WORKBOOK OVERVIEW

Glencoe Computers in the Medical Office is divided into four parts. The first, "Introduction to Computers in the Medical Office," covers the general flow of information in a medical office and the role that computers play. Instructors may wish to use the first part as a review or, if students have had other courses in computers, they may wish to start directly with Part 2. A test has been provided in the *Instructor's Manual* to determine the level of students' familiarity with computers.

Part 2, "MediSoft for Windows Training," teaches students how to start, input data, and use MediSoft to bill patients, file claims, record data, print reports, and schedule appointments. The sequence takes the student through MediSoft in a clear, concise manner. Each chapter includes a number of exercises that are to be done at the computer. These exercises give the student realistic experience using an administrative medical software program.

Part 3, "Applying Your Knowledge," completes the learning process by requiring the student to perform a series of tasks using MediSoft. Each task is an application of the knowledge required in the medical office.

At the end of the text/workbook, Part 4, a section of Source Documents, gives the student the data needed to complete the exercises. These forms, including patient information forms and superbills, are similar to those used in medical offices.

COMPUTER SUPPLIES AND EQUIPMENT

The Student Data Disk that comes with the text/workbook provides a base of case study information. Other equipment and supplies needed are as follows:

Pentium 200 processor or greater
32 MB RAM
Windows 95, 98, 2000, or NT
MediSoft Advanced Patient Accounting for Windows 5.66
Blank, formatted floppy diskette
Printer

MediSoft Advanced Patient Accounting for Windows is free to schools adopting *Glencoe Computers in the Medical Office*. Information on ordering and installing the software is located in the *Instructor's Manual* that accompanies the text/workbook.

CHAPTER STRUCTURE

At the beginning of each chapter, students are provided with a preview of what will be studied:

What You Need to Know   Describes the basic knowledge required in order to complete the chapter.

Objectives   Describes the primary areas of knowledge that can be acquired by studying the chapter and performing the exercises.

Key Terms   Presents an alphabetic list of important vocabulary terms found in the chapter. Key terms are printed in bold-faced type and defined when introduced in the text/workbook. Key term definitions also appear in the left margin of the page where they are first used.

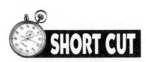

Throughout the instructional chapters, the narrative is supported by numerous figures and tables for reference. These instructional portions of the chapter include *Short Cut* and *Tip* features to enhance the learning experience (see icons in left margin). Computer exercises follow the portions of instructional material to reinforce what was just read.

Various types of testing are supplied in the *Chapter Review* at the end of each chapter in Parts 1 and 2. *Using Terminology* and *Checking Your Understanding* test the student's knowledge of the chapter's key terms and content. *Applying Knowledge* and *At the Computer* encourage the student to use critical thinking skills and apply practical knowledge using the computer.

SUPPLEMENTARY MATERIAL

An *Instructor's Manual* provides the instructor with answers to chapter exercises, answers to Chapter Review questions/exercises, teaching suggestions, SCANS and AAMA correlations, and information on ordering and installing MediSoft Advanced Patient Accounting for Windows software. The CD also contains the ExamView Pro test generator program.

ACKNOWLEDGMENTS

For insightful reviews, criticisms, helpful suggestions, and information, we would like to acknowledge the following:

Anne Conway
National Career Education
Citrus Heights, California

Christine E. Hetrick
Omega Institute
Pennsauken, New Jersey

Deborah Jones
Bryman School
Phoenix, Arizona

Debbie Kline
Eye Physicians and Surgeons
San Jose, California

Debra Peelor
Bidwell Training Center, Inc.
Pittsburgh, Pennsylvania

Nina Thierer
Ivy Tech State College
Fort Wayne, Indiana

Geraldine Todaro
Stark State College of Technology
Canton, Ohio

Introduction to Computers in the Medical Office

PART

1

Chapter 1
The Flow of Information in the Medical Office

Chapter 2
The Role of Computers in the Medical Office

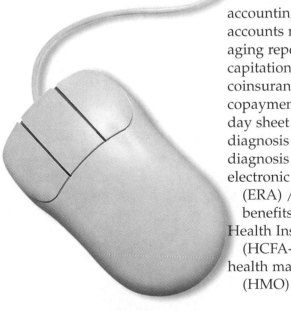

CHAPTER 1

The Flow of Information in the Medical Office

In this chapter, you will learn:

◆ The tasks that are performed on a regular basis in the medical office, including scheduling appointments, gathering and recording patient information, recording diagnoses and procedures, billing patients, filing insurance claims, reviewing and recording payments, and balancing the accounts.

◆ The different types of medical insurance.

◆ The steps involved in processing claims and collecting payments.

◆ The daily and monthly reports required to balance the practice's accounts receivable.

KEY TERMS

accounting cycle
accounts receivable (A/R)
aging reports
capitation
coinsurance
copayment
day sheet
diagnosis
diagnosis code
electronic remittance advice
  (ERA) / explanation of
  benefits (EOB)
Health Insurance Claim Form
  (HCFA-1500)
health maintenance organization
  (HMO)

indemnity plan
insurance carrier
managed care
patient information form
patient statement
policyholder
practice analysis report
preferred provider organization
  (PPO)
premiums
procedure code
procedures
providers
schedule of benefits
superbill
third-party payer

THE TASK CYCLE

policyholder an individual who has contracted with an insurance company for coverage.

insurance carrier a company that provides insurance coverage to individuals and/or groups.

premiums payments made to an insurance carrier by a policyholder for coverage.

providers physicians, hospitals, and other medical staff who provide medical services.

Most patients are covered by some type of medical insurance. Medical insurance is an agreement between a person, known as the **policyholder**, and an **insurance carrier**. Payments made to the carrier by the policyholder for insurance coverage are called **premiums**. In exchange for these payments, the carrier agrees to pay benefits for medical services. Medical services include care supplied by **providers**—hospitals, physicians, and other medical staff.

From a business standpoint, the key to the financial health of a medical practice is billing and collecting fees for services. Without a steady flow of money coming in, payroll cannot be met, supplies cannot be ordered, utility bills cannot be paid, and so on. To maintain a regular flow of income, certain tasks must be completed in a regular cycle and in a timely manner. These tasks include:

◆ Scheduling appointments

◆ Gathering and recording patient information

◆ Recording diagnoses and procedures

◆ Billing patients and filing insurance claims

◆ Reviewing and recording payments

◆ Balancing the accounts

SCHEDULING APPOINTMENTS

The cycle begins when a patient requests an appointment. New appointment requests are usually made by telephone; follow-up appointments are typically scheduled when the patient is at the front desk, having just seen the physician. When new patients phone for an appointment, they should be informed of the practice's policy regarding payment.

More and more medical offices are using computerized scheduling programs to keep track of patient appointments. If the individual requesting an appointment is an established patient of the practice, the medical office assistant searches for an available time slot that is suitable for the patient and books the appointment. If the individual is a new patient, basic information (such as the patient's name and phone number) is recorded when the appointment is booked. When the new patient arrives at the office for the appointment, additional information is collected. However, in some practices, this additional information is taken over the telephone at the time the appointment is made.

RECORDING PATIENT INFORMATION

The first time a patient visits the practice, a **patient information form** is completed (see Figure 1-1). The patient information form contains the personal, employment, and medical insurance information needed to file an insurance claim. This form is filed in the patient's medical record and is updated when the patient reports a change, such as a new address or a change in insurance carrier. Many offices ask patients to update these forms periodically to ensure that the information is current and accurate.

patient information form a document that contains personal, employment, and medical insurance information about a patient.

Some patient information forms also include miscellaneous information such as:

◆ Student status

◆ Patient allergies

◆ Referring physician

◆ Reason for visit

◆ Accident information, if appropriate

As shown in Figure 1-1 on page 6, the patient information form also has places for the patient's signature and for a parent's or guardian's signature if the patient is a minor, mentally incapacitated, or incompetent. One signature authorizes the insurance carrier or government program to send payments directly to the provider rather than to the patient. Patients are also asked to sign a release of information statement. This signature gives the medical office permission to release diagnosis and treatment information to the insurance company for the purpose of reimbursement for services provided by the physician.

RECORDING DIAGNOSES AND PROCEDURES

When the patient sees the physician, the complaint(s) and symptom(s) are entered in the patient's medical record. The **diagnosis**, which is the physician's opinion of the nature of the patient's illness or injury, as well as the **procedures**—the services performed—are recorded. Medications prescribed are also listed.

diagnosis a physician's opinion of the nature of an illness or injury.
procedures services performed by a provider.

When diagnoses and procedures are reported to insurance carriers, code numbers are used in place of narrative description. An electrocardiogram is not reported as an electrocardiogram or an ECG, but as 93000. Coding is a way of translating a description of a condition into a shorter, standardized code. Standardization allows information to be shared among physicians, office personnel, insurance carriers, and so on, without losing the precise meaning. Diagnosis and procedure codes are very precise. Insurance carriers base much of their claim approval decisions on the information indicated by diagnosis and procedure codes. Thus, the medical office staff member who does the coding must have specialized knowledge.

PATIENT INFORMATION FORM

THIS SECTION REFERS TO PATIENT ONLY			
Name:	Sex:	Marital status: ☐S ☐M ☐D ☐W	Birth date:
Address:	SS#:		
City: State: Zip:	Employer:		
Home phone:	Employer's address:		
Work phone:	City: State: Zip:		
Spouse's name:	Spouse's employer:		
Emergency contact:	Relationship: Phone #:		

FILL IN IF PATIENT IS A MINOR			
Parent/Guardian's name:	Sex:	Marital status: ☐S ☐M ☐D ☐W	Birth date:
Phone:	SS#:		
Address:	Employer:		
City: State: Zip:	Employer's address:		
Student status:	City: State: Zip:		

INSURANCE INFORMATION	
Primary insurance company:	Secondary insurance company:
Policyholder's name: Birth date:	Policyholder's name: Birth date:
Copayment: Price Code:	Copayment: Price Code:
Policy #: Group #:	Policy #: Group #:

OTHER INFORMATION	
Reason for visit:	Allergy to medication (list):
Name of referring physician:	If auto accident, list date and state in which it occurred:

(Patient's signature/Parent or guardian's signature) (Date)

Figure 1-1 **Sample patient information form.**

diagnosis code a standardized value used to describe a patient's illness, signs, and symptoms.

A patient's diagnosis is communicated to the insurance carrier as a **diagnosis code**, a code found in the *International Classification of Diseases* (ICD). Diagnostic codes provide insurance carriers with very specific information about the patient's specific illness(es), sign(s), and symptom(s). Errors in coding can delay the processing of claims and result in a reduced payment or the denial of a claim.

procedure code a standardized value that specifies which medical tests and procedures were performed.

Similarly, a **procedure code** is a standardized code that specifies which medical procedures and tests were performed. The most commonly used system of procedure codes is found in the *Current Procedural Terminology*, Fourth Edition, also known as the CPT. The CPT was developed to provide a standardized system to use when describing diagnostic procedures, such as an office visit to examine a patient, and therapeutic procedures, such as surgery and immunizations.

superbill a form listing procedures relevant to the specialty of a medical office, used to indicate what procedures were performed.

After entering diagnostic and procedural information in the patient's medical record, the physician completes a **superbill**, also known as an encounter form (see Figure 1-2 on page 8). The superbill lists procedures and codes relevant to the particular specialty of the medical office and may also include a list of typical diagnoses. It may provide a place for office visit charges and payments. The information on superbills should be checked on an annual basis to be sure that all current diagnoses and procedures and correct dates are listed as well as updated fees, if on the superbill.

BILLING PATIENTS AND FILING INSURANCE CLAIMS

During a typical day, dozens of patients visit the medical office. They have a variety of problems and needs, and they receive different services from the physician. When patients receive services from a medical practice, they either pay for services themselves, or the charges are submitted to their insurance company or government agency for payment. To receive payment, most medical practices must complete or produce documents for insurance carriers and patients. One kind of document is an insurance claim form. Although some private insurance carriers have specialized claim forms for their policyholders, most forms ask for the same basic information. Fortunately, most insurance carriers also accept a universal claim form called the **Health Insurance Claim Form**, approved by the American Medical Association and the Health Care Financing Administration. This form is commonly known as the **HCFA-1500**, or the HCFA (pronounced "hic-fa") form. As illustrated in Figure 1-3 on page 10, this form is used for governmental health programs and most private plans. Electronic claims are established in HCFA-1500 format.

Health Insurance Claim Form (HCFA-1500) a universal health insurance claim form used by governmental health programs and many private insurance carriers.

patient statement a document that informs the patient of the amount owed to the medical practice.

Sometimes charges are not covered by an insurance carrier and must be billed to the patient. The **patient statement** informs the patient of the amount owed for a specific visit. The patient statement lists all services performed, along with the associated charges. Most medical

Family Care Center
285 Stephenson Boulevard
Stephenson, OH 60089
(614)555-0000

Date: 12/8/03   **Name** _____

Chart Number _____   **Physician** _____

01	patient payment, cash		85651	erythrocyte sedimentation rate--non-auto
02	patient payment, check		86403	strep test, quick
03	insurance carrier payment		86585	tuberculosis, tine test
04	insurance company adjustment		86588	direct streptococcus screen
05	adjustment, patient		87072	culture by commercial kit, nonurine...
06	OhioCare HMO Charge - $10		87076	bacterial culture, anerobic, with GC...
07	OhioCare HMO Charge - $15		87086	urine culture and colony count
12011	simple suture--face--local anes.		90703	tetanus injection
29125	application of short arm splint; static		90782	injection with material, subcutaneous or
29425	application of short leg cast, walking		92516	facial nerve function studies
45378	colonoscopy--diagnostic		93000	Electrocardiogram--ECG with interpret...
45380	colonoscopy--with biopsy		93015	Treadmill stress test, with physician...
50390	aspiration of renal cyst by needle		96900	ultraviolet light treatment
71010	chest x-ray, single view, frontal		99070	supplies and materials provided
71020	chest x-ray, two views, frontal & lat...		99201	OF--new patient, problem focused
71030	chest x-ray, complete, four views		99202	OF--new patient, expanded
73070	elbow x-ray, AP and lateral views		99203	OF--new patient, detailed history and...
73090	forearm x-ray, AP and lateral views		99204	OF--new patient, comprehensive history..
73100	wrist x-ray, AP and lateral views		99205	OF--new patient, comprehensive history..
73510	hip x-ray, complete, two views		99211	OF--established patient, minimal
73600	ankle x-ray, AP and lateral views		99212	OF--established patient, problem focused
80019	19 clinical chemistry tests		99213	OF--established patient, expanded
80061	lipid panel		99214	OF--established patient, detailed...
82270	blood screening, occult; feces		99215	OF--established patient, comprehensive..
82947	glucose screening--quantitative		99394	established patient, adolescent, per...
82951	glucose tolerance test, three specimens		99396	established patient, 40-64 years, per...
83718	HDL cholesterol			
84478	triglycerides test			
85007	manual differential WBC			
85022	hemogram, automated, and manual...			

Payments _____   **Remarks** _____

Diagnosis _____   _____

Figure 1-2 **Sample superbill.**

practices have a regular schedule, perhaps daily or weekly, for submitting claims to insurance carriers. For example, some practices bill half the patients on the fifteenth of the month and the other half on the thirtieth.

Overview of Medical Insurance

There are a wide variety of medical insurance plans in the United States. Many people are covered by group policies, often through their employers. Other people, such as those who are self-employed, have individual plans. Insurance coverage may be supplied by a private company, such as Aetna, or by a government plan. Some of the most common government plans in effect in the United States are:

◆ **Medicare** Medicare is a federal health plan that covers persons aged 65 and over, people with disabilities, and dependent widows.

◆ **Medicaid** People with low incomes who cannot afford medical care are covered by Medicaid, which is cosponsored by federal and state governments. Qualifications and benefits vary by state.

◆ **TRICARE** TRICARE is a government program that covers medical expenses for dependents of active duty members of the uniformed services and for retired military personnel. Formerly known as CHAMPUS, it also covers dependents of military personnel who were killed while on active duty.

◆ **CHAMPVA** The Civilian Health and Medical Program of the Veterans Administration is for veterans with permanent service-related disabilities and their dependents. It also covers surviving spouses and dependent children of veterans who died from service-related disabilities.

◆ **Workers' Compensation** People with job-related illnesses or injuries are covered under workers' compensation insurance. Workers' compensation benefits vary according to state law.

third-party payer a term used to describe an insurance carrier in the context of the physician's and the patient's relationship.

Whether private company or government program, the insurance carrier is called a **third-party payer**. The primary relationship is between the physician and the patient. The insurance carrier is the third party.

indemnity plan an insurance plan in which policyholders are reimbursed for health care costs.

schedule of benefits in an insurance policy, a listing of services covered and the amount of coverage.

Different types of insurance plans can be purchased. In an **indemnity plan**, policyholders are paid back for costs for health care due to illnesses and accidents. Under an indemnity plan, the **schedule of benefits** in the policy lists the services that are covered and the amounts that are paid. The benefit may be for all or part of the charges. For example, the schedule of benefits may indicate that 80 percent of charges for surgery performed in a hospital are covered. The policy-

APPROVED OMB-0938-0008

CARRIER

HEALTH INSURANCE CLAIM FORM

PICA [ ][ ]

[ ][ ] PICA

1. MEDICARE   MEDICAID   CHAMPUS   CHAMPVA   GROUP   FECA   OTHER   1a. INSURED'S I.D. NUMBER   (FOR PROGRAM IN ITEM 1)
   [ ] (Medicare #)   [ ] (Medicaid #)   [ ] (Sponsor's SSN)   [ ] (VA File #)   [ ] HEALTH PLAN   [ ] BLK LUNG   [ ] (ID)
      (SSN or ID)   (SSN)

2. PATIENT'S NAME (Last Name, First Name, Middle Initial)   3. PATIENT'S BIRTH DATE   SEX   4. INSURED'S NAME (Last Name, First Name, Middle Initial)
                                    MM   DD   YY   M [ ]   F [ ]

5. PATIENT'S ADDRESS (No., Street)   6. PATIENT RELATIONSHIP TO INSURED   7. INSURED'S ADDRESS (No., Street)
                                  Self [ ]   Spouse [ ]   Child [ ]   Other [ ]

CITY   STATE   8. PATIENT STATUS   CITY   STATE
                                 Single [ ]   Married [ ]   Other [ ]

ZIP CODE   TELEPHONE (Include Area Code)   ZIP CODE   TELEPHONE (INCLUDE AREA CODE)
               (   )   Employed [ ]   Full-Time [ ]   Part-Time [ ]   (   )
                                     Student   Student

9. OTHER INSURED'S NAME (Last Name, First Name, Middle Initial)   10. IS PATIENT'S CONDITION RELATED TO: 11. INSURED'S POLICY GROUP OR FECA NUMBER

a. OTHER INSURED'S POLICY OR GROUP NUMBER   a. EMPLOYMENT? (CURRENT OR PREVIOUS)   a. INSURED'S DATE OF BIRTH   SEX
                                 [ ] YES   [ ] NO   MM   DD   YY   M [ ]   F [ ]

b. OTHER INSURED'S DATE OF BIRTH   SEX   b. AUTO ACCIDENT?   PLACE (State)   b. EMPLOYER'S NAME OR SCHOOL NAME
  MM   DD   YY   M [ ]   F [ ]   [ ] YES   [ ] NO

c. EMPLOYER'S NAME OR SCHOOL NAME   c. OTHER ACCIDENT?   c. INSURANCE PLAN NAME OR PROGRAM NAME
                                 [ ] YES   [ ] NO

d. INSURANCE PLAN NAME OR PROGRAM NAME   10d. RESERVED FOR LOCAL USE   d. IS THERE ANOTHER HEALTH BENEFIT PLAN?
                                                [ ] YES   [ ] NO   **If yes**, return to and complete item 9 a-d.

READ BACK OF FORM BEFORE COMPLETING & SIGNING THIS FORM.

12. PATIENT'S OR AUTHORIZED PERSON'S SIGNATURE I authorize the release of any medical or other information necessary to process this claim. I also request payment of government benefits either to myself or to the party who accepts assignment below.

SIGNED _____ DATE _____

13. INSURED'S OR AUTHORIZED PERSON'S SIGNATURE I authorize payment of medical benefits to the undersigned physician or supplier for services described below.

SIGNED _____

14. DATE OF CURRENT: ILLNESS (First symptom) OR   15. IF PATIENT HAS HAD SAME OR SIMILAR ILLNESS,   16. DATES PATIENT UNABLE TO WORK IN CURRENT OCCUPATION
  MM   DD   YY   ◀ INJURY (Accident) OR   GIVE FIRST DATE   MM   DD   YY   FROM MM   DD   YY   TO   MM   DD   YY
              PREGNANCY (LMP)

17. NAME OF REFERRING PHYSICIAN OR OTHER SOURCE   17a. I.D. NUMBER OF REFERRING PHYSICIAN   18. HOSPITALIZATION DATES RELATED TO CURRENT SERVICES
                                                 FROM MM   DD   YY   TO   MM   DD   YY

19. RESERVED FOR LOCAL USE   20. OUTSIDE LAB? $ CHARGES
                                                 [ ] YES   [ ] NO

21. DIAGNOSIS OR NATURE OF ILLNESS OR INJURY. (RELATE ITEMS 1,2,3, OR 4 TO ITEM 24E BY LINE)   22. MEDICAID RESUBMISSION
                                                  CODE   ORIGINAL REF. NO.

1. |___.___   3. |___.___

                                               23. PRIOR AUTHORIZATION NUMBER

2. |___.___   4. |___.___

24. A		B	C	D		E	F	G	H	I	J	K
DATE(S) OF SERVICE		Place of Service	Type of Service	PROCEDURES, SERVICES, OR SUPPLIES (Explain Unusual Circumstances)		DIAGNOSIS CODE	$ CHARGES	DAYS OR UNITS	EPSDT Family Plan	EMG	COB	RESERVED FOR LOCAL USE
From MM DD YY	To MM DD YY			CPT/HCPCS	MODIFIER							
1												
2												
3												
4												
5												
6												

25. FEDERAL TAX I.D. NUMBER   SSN EIN   26. PATIENT'S ACCOUNT NO.   27. ACCEPT ASSIGNMENT?   28. TOTAL CHARGE   29. AMOUNT PAID   30. BALANCE DUE
                                         (For govt. claims, see back)   [ ] YES   [ ] NO $ $ $

31. SIGNATURE OF PHYSICIAN OR SUPPLIER INCLUDING DEGREES OR CREDENTIALS (I certify that the statements on the reverse apply to this bill and are made a part thereof.)   32. NAME AND ADDRESS OF FACILITY WHERE SERVICES WERE RENDERED (if other than home or office)   33. PHYSICIAN'S OR SUPPLIER'S NAME, ADDRESS, ZIP CODE & TELEPHONE NO.

SIGNED _____ DATE _____   PIN# _____ GRP# _____

PATIENT AND INSURED INFORMATION   PHYSICIAN OR SUPPLIER INFORMATION

(APPROVED BY AMA COUNCIL ON MEDICAL SERVICE 8/88)   **PLEASE PRINT OR TYPE**   FORM HCFA-1500 (12-90)
                                                       FORM OWCP-1500   FORM RRB-1500

Figure 1-3 Health Insurance Claim Form (HCFA-1500).

coinsurance *a type of insurance plan in which the patient is responsible for a percentage of the charges.*

managed care *a type of insurance in which the insurance carrier is responsible for the financing and the delivery of health care.*

preferred provider organization (PPO) *a type of managed care system in which patients pay fixed rates at regular intervals.*

health maintenance organization (HMO) *a type of managed care system in which patients pay fixed rates at regular intervals.*

copayment *a small fixed fee paid by the patient at the time of an office visit.*

capitation *a type of managed care system in which patients pay fixed rates at regular intervals.*

holder is responsible for paying the other 20 percent. This amount—the portion of charges that an insured person must pay for health care services—is known as **coinsurance**.

Another type of insurance system is **managed care**. Managed care was introduced in the mid-1980s as a way of supervising health care to ensure that patients get the necessary care in the most appropriate, cost-effective setting. A managed care company is responsible for both the financing and the delivery of health care to its policyholders. The company signs up providers who agree to supply services for a fixed fee. The providers do not set the fees. Instead, the fees are set by the company or government agency that has a contract with the providers.

The most common type of managed care program is a **preferred provider organization (PPO)**. A PPO is a network of health care providers who agree to perform services for plan members at discounted fees. In most plans, members may receive care from providers outside the network for a higher cost.

Another common type of managed care system is a **health maintenance organization (HMO)**. In an HMO, patients pay fixed rates at regular intervals, such as monthly. In some HMOs, patients pay a **copayment**—a small fixed fee, such as $10, at the time of the office visit. In HMOs, patients must choose from a specific group of physicians and hospitals for their medical care.

In some managed care plans, physicians are paid a fixed amount per month to provide necessary, contracted services to patients who are plan members. This fixed prepayment is referred to as **capitation**. The rate the physician is paid is based on several factors, including the number of plan members, and their age and gender. The capitated rate is paid to the physician even if the physician does not provide any medical services to the patient during the time period covered by the payment. Similarly, the physician receives the same capitated rate if a patient is treated more than once during the time period.

Processing Claims

For an insurance carrier to pay a claim, certain information about the patient must be shared. For example, the insurance carrier needs to know the physician's assessment of the patient's condition—the patient's diagnosis—and the procedures the physician performed while the patient was in the office. The date of the visit and the location of the visit (such as physician's office or hospital) must be posted. The insurance carrier also requires basic information about the physician providing the treatment, including the provider's name and/or provider identification number. There may be a group number and an individual identification number for a provider who is part of a group practice.

The information needed to create a claim is found on the patient information form and the superbill. Most insurance claims are submitted electronically by transferring information from a computer in the provider's office to a computer at the insurance company. In some instances, such as when an attachment is required, paper forms are filed. Some offices use a clearinghouse for claims filed electronically.

When the claim is received by the insurance carrier, it is reviewed and processed. If the patient's insurance is an indemnity plan, the insurance company compares the fees to the schedule of benefits in the patient's policy and determines the amount of benefit to be paid. If the patient's insurance coverage is a managed care plan, the insurance company pays a contracted fee to the provider, and the patient pays the copayment directly to the provider.

REVIEWING AND RECORDING PAYMENTS

electronic remittance advice (ERA) / explanation of benefits (EOB) a document from an insurance carrier that lists the amount of a benefit and explains how it was determined.

After the amount of the benefit is determined, the insurance carrier issues a payment. At the same time, it issues an **electronic remittance advice (ERA)**, or **explanation of benefits (EOB)**. An ERA is used with electronic claims, while an EOB is sent when a paper claim is submitted. An ERA or EOB indicates how the amount of benefit was determined (see Figure 1-4). The insurance company sends the payment to the physician or to the policyholder to whom it is owed.

When the ERA arrives at the physician's office, it is reviewed for accuracy. If an error is found, a request for a review of the claim must be filed with the carrier. If a check is enclosed, the amount of the payment from the insurance carrier is recorded. In some cases, the patient is billed for an outstanding balance. In other circumstances, an account adjustment is made.

BALANCING THE ACCOUNTS

accounting cycle the flow of financial transactions in a business.

accounts receivable (A/R) monies that are flowing in to a business.

day sheet a report that lists all transactions for a single day.

The **accounting cycle** is the flow of financial transactions in a business—from making a sale to collecting payment for the goods or services delivered. In a medical practice, this is the cycle from seeing and treating the patient to receiving payments for services provided.

Accounting software can be used to track **accounts receivable (A/R)** —monies that are coming in to the practice—and to produce financial reports. Reports are usually created at the end of each day and at the end of the month, quarter, and year. At the end of each day, a report is generated that lists all charges, payments, and adjustments entered during that day. This report is known as a **day sheet**. To balance out a day, transactions listed on superbills (charges and payments) and totals from deposit tickets are compared against the computer-generated day sheet.

CUSTOMER'S EXPLANATION OF BENEFITS

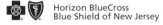 Horizon BlueCross
Blue Shield of New Jersey

An Independent Licensee of the Blue Cross and Blue Shield Association

THIS IS NOT A BILL RETAIN FOR YOUR RECORDS

PAGE 1 OF 2

CUSTOMER'S NAME: SUSAN
ID NUMBER: 140385527
PATIENT'S NAME: SUSAN

COVERAGE: HORIZON BCBS OF NJ

CONSUMER DIVISION

CLAIM NUMBER: 7970860005450000
CLAIM RECEIVED: 03/27/2004
CLAIM FINALIZED: 04/02/2004
CHECK NUMBER: 0005878547

MEDICARE SURGICAL/MAJOR MEDICAL
CLAIM SUMMARY

CHARGES FOR THIS CLAIM .... $ 1,500.00
AMOUNT OF CUSTOMER BALANCE REMAINING............... $ 870.79
BENEFITS PAID TO SUSAN BALE .... $ 630.00

DO NOT SUBMIT A SEPARATE MAJOR MEDICAL CLAIM FORM
THIS CLAIM HAS BEEN PROCESSED UNDER YOUR MEDICAL-SURGICAL AND MAJOR MEDICAL CONTRACTS

★ ★ ★ ★ FOR A DETAILED SUMMARY OF YOUR CLAIM PLEASE SEE REVERSE ★ ★ ★ ★

CLAIM DETAIL
PAGE 2 OF 2

PATIENT'S NAME: SUSAN   IDENTIFICATION NUMBER : 140385527   CLAIM NUMBER: 7970860005450000

PROVIDER NAME		1	2	3	4	5	6	7	8	9
TYPE OF SERVICE - PLACE OF SERVICE	DATE OF SERVICE FROM TO	CHARGE AMOUNT	OTHER INS PAYMENT	NOT COVERED AMOUNT	ELIGIBLE AMOUNT	DEDUCT-IBLE	CO-INS. / CO-PAY	BENEFIT AMOUNT	CUSTOMER BALANCE	MSG CODES
WESTFIELD OB GYN ASSOCIATES										
ASST SURG -INPATIENT	03/13/04 03/13/04	1500.00			900.00		270.00	630.00		A
	MAJOR MEDICAL	1500.00						0.00	870.00	
TOTALS		1500.00			900.00		270.00	630.00	870.00	
				MESSAGES						

CRP027 (12-97) Rev

* SUSAN HAS SATISFIED $ 1,000.00 OF HER DEDUCTIBLE FOR THE PERIOD 01-01-2004 TO 12-31-2004. (D055)

A-PROVIDER'S CHARGES EXCEED OUR ALLOWED AMOUNT FOR THIS SERVICE. THIS EXCESS AMOUNT, INCLUDED IN THE CUSTOMER
   BALANCE COLUMN, IS YOUR LIABILITY. (D223)

Figure 1-4 **Sample explanation of benefits statement.**

practice analysis report a document from an insurance carrier that lists the amount of a benefit and explains how it was determined.

At the end of the month, a **practice analysis report** summarizes the financial activity of the entire month. This reports lists charges, payments, and adjustments and the total accounts receivable for the month. It is possible to balance out the month by taking all the day sheets for the month, totaling the charges, payments, and adjustments, and then comparing the totals to the amounts listed on the practice analysis report.

aging reports a document from an insurance carrier that lists the amount of a benefit and explains how it was determined.

It is also good practice to print **aging reports** on a monthly basis. Aging reports list the outstanding balances owed to the practice by insurance companies or patients. There are also reports that provide current information on the status of patient and insurance billing. Monthly review of this report can alert the billing staff to accounts that require action to collect the amount due. In addition to these reports, most accounting programs provide other useful report tools that offer a clear picture of the practice's financial health at any point in time. Timely printing of reports also helps the office staff meet claim filing deadlines and collect unpaid insurance payments.

USING TERMINOLOGY

Match the terms on the left with the definitions on the right.

_____ 1. accounting cycle

_____ 2. accounts receivable (A/R)

_____ 3. aging report

_____ 4. capitation

_____ 5. coinsurance

_____ 6. copayment

_____ 7. day sheet

_____ 8. diagnosis

_____ 9. diagnosis code (ICD)

_____ 10. electronic remittance advice (ERA) / explanation of benefits (EOB)

_____ 11. health maintenance organization (HMO)

_____ 12. indemnity plan

_____ 13. insurance carrier

_____ 14. Health Insurance Claim Form (HCFA-1500)

a. A document from an insurance carrier that lists the amount of a benefit and explains how it was determined.

b. A universal health insurance claim form used by governmental health programs and many private insurance carriers.

c. A document that contains personal, employment, and medical insurance information about a patient.

d. A document that informs the patient of the amount owed to the medical practice after the insurance carrier has paid its portion of the bill.

e. A form listing procedures relevant to the specialty of a medical office, used to indicate what procedures were performed.

f. In an insurance policy, a listing of services covered and the amount of coverage.

g. A term used to describe an insurance carrier in the context of the physician's and the patient's relationship.

h. Services performed by a provider.

i. A report that lists outstanding balances owed to the practice.

j. An individual who has contracted with an insurance company for coverage.

k. Payments made to an insurance carrier by a policyholder for coverage.

l. A fixed amount that is paid to physicians in advance to provide necessary services to patients.

m. A type of insurance in which the carrier is responsible for the financing and the delivery of health care.

n. A term used to describe money coming in to a business.

_____ **15.** managed care

_____ **16.** patient information form

_____ **17.** patient statement

_____ **18.** policyholder

_____ **19.** practice analysis report

_____ **20.** preferred provider organization (PPO)

_____ **21.** premiums

_____ **22.** procedure code (CPT)

_____ **23.** procedures

_____ **24.** providers

_____ **25.** schedule of benefits

_____ **26.** superbill

_____ **27.** third party payer

o. A physician's opinion of the nature of an illness or injury.

p. A standardized value used to describe a patient's illness, signs, and symptoms.

q. An insurance plan in which policyholders are reimbursed for health care costs.

r. Under an insurance plan, the portion or percentage of the charges that the patient is responsible for paying.

s. A network of health care providers who agree to provide services to plan members at a discounted fee.

t. A report that summarizes the financial activity of a practice for a period of time, such as a month or year.

u. A standardized value that specifies which medical tests and procedures were performed.

v. Physicians, hospitals, and other medical staff who provide medical services.

w. A company that provides insurance coverage to individuals and/or groups.

x. A report that summarizes the financial activity of a practice for a single day.

y. A type of managed care system in which patients pay fixed rates at regular intervals.

z. A small fixed fee paid by the patient at the time of an office visit.

aa. The flow of financial transactions in a business.

CHECKING YOUR UNDERSTANDING

Write "T" or "F" in the blank to indicate whether you think the statement is true or false.

_____ **28.** Many patient information forms contain a place for the patient to sign to authorize the patient's insurance carrier to send payments directly to a provider.

_____ **29.** Insurance carriers look closely at procedure and diagnosis codes when making claim approval decisions.

_____ **30.** Coinsurance refers to a small fixed fee that must be paid by the patient at the time of an office visit.

_____ **31.** To receive payment for services, most medical offices must create two documents (either paper or electronic)—a patient statement and an insurance claim.

Answer the question below in the space provided.

32. List the six basic categories of administrative tasks in a medical office.

_____

_____

_____

_____

_____

_____

Choose the best answer.

_____ **33.** A patient information form contains information such as name, address, employer, and:
a. diagnosis code
b. insurance coverage information
c. charges for procedures performed

_____ **34.** A health maintenance organization (HMO) is one example of:
a. an indemnity plan
b. a government plan
c. a managed care plan

_____ **35.** In a managed care plan, a _____ is collected from the patient at the office visit.
    a. deductible
    b. patient statement
    c. copayment

_____ **36.** The most commonly used system of procedure codes is found in the:
    a. CPT
    b. ICD
    c. HCFA-1500

_____ **37.** Information about a patient's medical procedures that is needed to create an insurance claim is found on the:
    a. remittance advice
    b. patient statement
    c. superbill

CHAPTER 2

The Role of Computers in the Medical Office

KEY TERMS

audit/edit report
clearinghouse
database
e-commerce
electronic funds transfer (EFT)

electronic media claim (EMC)
electronic medical records (EMR)
health informatics
walkout receipt

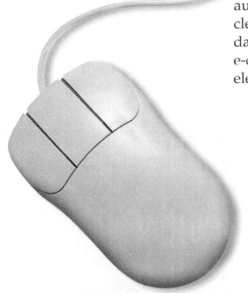

INTRODUCTION

In the past, most of the administrative work carried out in the medical office involved paper. Appointments were recorded in scheduling books, insurance claims were printed on paper forms, physicians' schedules were often prepared with handwritten notes, and so on. All this paper had to be filed and stored.

health informatics the electronic collection and management of health care information.

database a collection of related facts.

Today, the trend is to use computers for the storage, retrieval, and transmission of health information. **Health informatics** refers to the electronic collection and management of health data and information. Most medical offices use computers to perform a variety of administrative tasks. Information is entered into computer programs that are structured as a collection of related facts called a **database**. A medical office computer database stores information about providers, patients, insurance carriers, procedure codes, diagnosis codes, charges, and payments. Computers are used to verify insurance eligibility, produce insurance claims, store and retrieve medical records, create financial reports, accept electronic payments, schedule appointments, handle payroll, prepare referral letters, and more. Computer literacy has become a basic requirement for employment in an administrative position in a medical office.

A TYPICAL DAY IN A COMPUTERIZED MEDICAL OFFICE

To understand the role that computers play in today's medical office, consider a typical day in a computerized medical office. At the beginning of each day, the computer is used to print a listing of all appointments for that day for each physician in the office (see Figure 2-1). New appointments are booked during the day using an electronic scheduling program. As each patient arrives, new or revised data on patient information forms, such as patients' addresses, insurance plans, allergies, and so on, are keyed into the computer. Insurance eligibility is verified over the Internet or directly with the carrier via modem.

walkout receipt a document listing charges and payments that is given to a patient after an office visit.

As the physicians see patients, diagnoses and procedures are recorded on computer-generated superbills. Some physicians record clinical notes in the examining room; the notes are transferred to the computer later. When an office visit is completed, information from the superbill is entered into the computerized billing program. If the patient has made a payment, the computer prints a **walkout receipt**, which lists the charges and the amount paid by the patient (see Figure 2-2 on page 22).

Family Care Center   **Monday, November 15, 2004**

Rudner, John

Time	Name	Phone	Length	Notes
	Chart Number	Resource	Procedure	Repeat Description
1:15p				
1:30p				
1:45p	Lisa Green	(614)555-3606	45 99203	
2:00p				
2:15p				
2:30p	Bell, Herbert BELLHER0	(614)030-1111	60	
2:45p				
3:00p				
3:15p				
3:30p	Fitzwilliams, John FITZWJO0	(614)002-1111	30	
3:45p				
4:00p	Patterson, Leila PATTELE0	(614)666-0099	15	
4:15p	Klein, Randall KLEINRA0	(614)022-2693	30	
4:30p				
4:45p				

Figure 2-1 *Sample computerized appointment schedule for a physician (MediSoft).*

Family Care Center

285 Stephenson Boulevard
Stephenson, OH 60089
(614)555-0000

Page: 1

7/12/2004

Patient:	Paul Ramos	Diagnosis:	1.	706.1	severe acne
	39 Locust Avenue		2.		
	Stephenson, OH 60089		3.		
			4.		

Chart #: RAMOSPA0

Case #: 13

Instructions: Complete the patient information portion of your own insurance claim form. Attach this bill, signed and dated, and all other bills pertaining to the claim. If you have a deductible policy, hold your claim forms until you have met your deductible. Mail directly to your insurance carrier.

Date	Description	Procedure	Modify	DX	Units	Charge
7/12/2004	OF--new patient, problem focused	99201		1	1	32.00
7/12/2004	ultraviolet light treatment	96900		1	1	15.00
7/12/2004	East Ohio PPO Copayment	EAPCOPAY			1	-15.00

Provider Information

Provider Name:	John Rudner MD
License:	84701
Insurance PIN:	
SSN or EIN:	339-67-5000

Total Charges:	$ 47.00
Total Payments:	-$ 15.00
Total Adjustments:	$ 0.00
Total Due This Visit:	**$ 32.00**
Total Account Balance:	$ 14.00

Assign and Release: I hereby authorize payment of medical benefits to this physician for the services described above. I also authorize the release of any information necessary to process this claim.

Patient Signature: _____ Date: _____

Figure 2-2 **Sample walkout receipt (MediSoft).**

Insurance claims are created in a billing program, and the medical office assistant uses the computer to electronically transmit claims to insurance carriers for payment or to print paper claims. Once the claim has been processed by the insurance company, payment is transmitted electronically to the practice's bank account or mailed to the practice. Claim information is also sent from the carrier to the practice, and recorded in the computer by the billing specialist. The patient is then billed for any remaining balance. At the end of the day, reports are printed showing the daily activity of the practice—the number of patient visits, the diagnosis and procedure codes used, the fees charged, and the payments received. At the end of the month, financial reports are created and analyzed.

MEDICAL OFFICE APPLICATIONS

The tasks listed in Table 2-1 are performed on a regular basis in most medical offices. In each instance, the task can be completed more efficiently with the use of a specialized computer application. Each computer application is discussed separately in the following section of the chapter.

Table 2-1 Computer Applications in a Medical Office

Task	Computer Application
Scheduling	Scheduling application: Scheduling appointments and producing recall notices
Medical Records	Electronic medical records application: Recording and storing chart notes, test results, medication, etc.
Accounting	Billing/accounting application: Entering transactions, creating and processing claims, billing patients, receiving electronic payments, generating financial reports
Correspondence	E-mail: Sending referral letters, patient recall notices, etc.
Inventory/Supplies	E-commerce: Ordering office and medical supplies and equipment

SCHEDULING Computers are often used to keep track of physicians' schedules. Appointments can easily be canceled, moved to a different day, and so on. Computers can also print a daily list of appointments for each provider in the practice. Recurring appointments can be booked for future dates, such as once a week for the next six weeks. In addition, patient recall appointment notices can be generated on a timely basis.

One of the major advantages of computerized scheduling is the ability to easily locate scheduled appointments. For example, suppose a patient calls to ask when his or her next appointment is scheduled. Instead of searching page by page in a paper schedule book, the medical office assistant enters the patient's name in a search box, and the computer locates the appointment. Computer scheduling also simplifies the entry of repeated appointments. Rather than looking through an appointment book for acceptable dates and times, the computer performs the search and displays available dates and times. Computer scheduling programs are also used to store information about time reserved for surgeries, seminars, lunches, days off, and so on.

MEDICAL RECORDS

electronic medical records
patient medical records that are stored in a computer instead of on paper.

Electronic medical records (EMR) are patient medical records that are stored in a computer instead of on paper. EMR programs are being implemented in medical offices because they offer substantial benefits to the practice. One of the most important aspects of an electronic medical record is instant access to data from any location. A patient's entire medical history, including physician notes, surgeries, test results, X rays, lab work, medications prescribed, progress notes, and so on, is all part of an electronic medical record.

More and more, patient data is being transmitted electronically. For example, the results of blood work completed by an outside lab can be sent to the physician's office via computer. An EMR program is capable of receiving this electronic information and storing it in the appropriate patient record. Some physicians enter clinical notes on a portable handheld device, and the notes are later transferred to the EMR.

Once clinical information is entered into the computer, it can be transmitted to another computer with just a few commands. This can be especially helpful in emergency situations. For example, suppose a patient who had coronary bypass surgery eight weeks ago is admitted to the hospital complaining of chest pain today. The computer at the physician's office could transmit clinical information on the patient's condition to a computer at the hospital in just seconds. Results of prior tests and lab work, such as electrocardiograms, could be sent, as well as a list of medication currently taken by the patient. In a case such as this, where time is critical, the computer can be a lifesaving device.

Storing patient records on the computer also brings up the issue of computer security and the confidentiality of patient records. Everyone working in a medical office is charged with the responsibility of maintaining patient confidentiality. Many states have laws that protect a patient's privacy. If the patient's medical record is stored on the computer, who should have access to that data? How will the data be safeguarded so the information does not end up where it does not belong?

In response to questions such as these, organizations have developed guidelines for computer security. As one security measure, many medical offices assign passwords to individuals who have access to computer files, thereby limiting access to data stored on the computer. Access is granted on an as-needed basis. For example, the individual responsible for scheduling may not be able to access medical records or billing data. On the other hand, the physicians and several others (such as the practice manager) most likely have access to all databases.

As additional security, computer programs keep track of data entry and create an audit trail. When new information is entered or existing data is changed, a log is created to record the time and date of the entry as well as the name of the computer operator. This log is stored and may be reviewed by the practice manager on a regular basis to detect irregularities. In addition, if an error has been made, the program lists the name of the operator and the date the information was entered.

ACCOUNTING

Like other businesses, medical offices keep track of accounts receivable, or payments coming in from patients and insurance carriers, and accounts payable, or amounts owed to suppliers and staff. Keeping accurate financial records is critical to a practice's survival. Not only are accurate records needed to meet financial obligations, but they are also required for tax reporting purposes. And, as in any business, accurate financial reports let management know whether the medical office is profitable.

Computerized accounting programs perform the tasks that were accomplished manually in the past. Medical offices may use different computerized accounting systems to keep track of their finances, but all accounting systems require certain types of information:

Patient Data Personal information about the patient, as well as information on the patient's insurance coverage, is extracted from the program's patient database.

Transaction Data Transaction information is taken from the superbill and keyed into the computer program. It includes the date of the visit, diagnosis and procedures codes, lab work, medications prescribed, and payments.

From these sources of information, patient statements are generated, insurance claims are created, and reports on the financial health of the practice are produced.

Insurance Claims

One of the major uses of computer technology in the medical office is to create insurance claims. A computerized system automatically generates completed insurance forms. The forms can be printed or transmitted electronically. By comparison, if a manual system is used, the medical office assistant must first compile all the needed resources and then key all the data on the claim form. This process takes longer and is more likely to create processing errors.

MediSoft, the computerized health care billing system used in *Computers in the Medical Office*, is one example of a computer program used in the medical office to process insurance claims. Processing information to create completed insurance claim forms is one of the main functions of programs such as MediSoft. Three major steps are followed to create insurance claims using MediSoft: (1) setting up the practice, (2) entering transaction information, and (3) creating and transmitting the completed insurance claim form.

Before a medical practice opens its doors to patients, a lot of preparation must be done. Equipment, supplies, staff, and procedures all need to be readied. Similarly, before MediSoft is used to store information about patients and their visits, basic facts about the practice itself are entered. Often a computer consultant or an accountant helps set up MediSoft's records about the practice. Then the provider database is entered, including descriptions of each physician's office hours and facts about referring physicians and lab services. Finally, the insurance carrier database is entered. It contains information about the carriers that most patients use. Each database in MediSoft is linked, or related, to each of the others by having at least one fact in common.

When a patient visits a physician, information about the visit is collected on the patient information form and the superbill. After analyzing and checking the data, the medical office assistant enters each element in the computer program. A new record must be created for a new patient, and established patients' information may need to be updated. Next, the appropriate insurance carrier for the visit is selected. Then, the purposes of the visit, the diagnosis codes, and the procedure codes are entered, with the appropriate charges.

When all transaction information has been entered and checked, the medical office assistant issues the command to MediSoft to create an insurance claim form. The format for the claim—either the HCFA-1500 or a specialized claim form—is also designated. MediSoft then organizes the necessary databases and selects the data from each database as needed to produce a complete claim form. The program follows the instructions to print or transmit the form electronically to the designated receiver.

An **electronic media claim (EMC)** is an insurance claim that is sent by a computer over a telephone line using a modem. Electronic claim filing has several advantages. First, it is faster to file and process claims electronically than to fill out and process paper forms, and it requires fewer staff members. In addition, it costs less to file electronically; the costs of paper forms, envelopes, and postage are much higher than the costs of transmission over phone lines. Also, chances of error or omission are reduced because information is entered once, not twice. In the case of paper forms, information also has to be entered into the insurance company's computer when the forms arrive by mail.

Usually, EMCs are paid faster than paper claims. For example, Medicare pays electronic claims in about half the time it takes for paper claims to be paid. Another advantage for the provider of submitting an EMC is **electronic funds transfer (EFT)**. This capability, which is an optional part of most EMC processing systems, allows for payments to be deposited directly into the provider's bank account. Many carriers' systems are also set up to provide electronic remittance advice (ERA). An ERA is much faster than one sent through the mail, since the information is transmitted directly to the provider's computer by modem. Questions can thus be resolved faster, improving the provider's receipt of payment.

Problems with EMCs usually result when transmission failures occur as a result of power outages. Transmission problems may also result from the breakdown of computer equipment. In these cases, the remedy is to retransmit missing claims after the problem is solved.

Electronic media claims can be sent directly to an insurance carrier, or they can be sent to a **clearinghouse**. A clearinghouse is a service bureau that collects electronic insurance claims from many different medical practices and forwards the claims to the appropriate insurance carriers (see Figure 2-3 on page 28). Some insurance carriers who receive insurance claims electronically require information to be formatted in a certain way. Clearinghouses translate claim data to fit the setup of each carrier's claims processing department. Because of this factor, many medical practices choose to use a clearinghouse instead of transmitting claims directly to insurance carriers.

When a clearinghouse receives claims, it checks to see that all necessary information is included. An **audit/edit report** is used to communicate problems that need to be corrected to the medical office (see Figure 2-4 on page 29). This reduces the number of claim rejections by insurance carriers and speeds the processing and payment of claims.

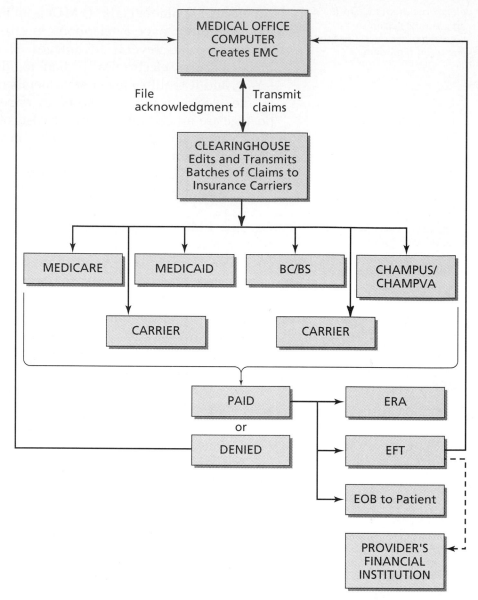

Figure 2-3 **Example of EMC flow using a clearinghouse (courtesy of The Computer Place/MediSoft).**

CORRESPONDENCE

Like other businesses, medical offices use computers to produce written correspondence, reports, forms, and other documents. These documents can be printed and mailed, or they can be sent via e-mail. A common use of e-mail is managed care referral letters. Correspondence that normally took several days can now be transmitted in a matter of seconds. Documents are stored electronically, which greatly reduces the amount of storage space required. Once again, practices that use e-mail for this purpose must have security measures in place to safeguard patient confidentiality.

INVENTORY/ SUPPLIES

The Internet is being used by some practices to order medical supplies and equipment. **E-commerce**—the exchange of funds over the Internet—allows offices to purchase supplies online at a discount

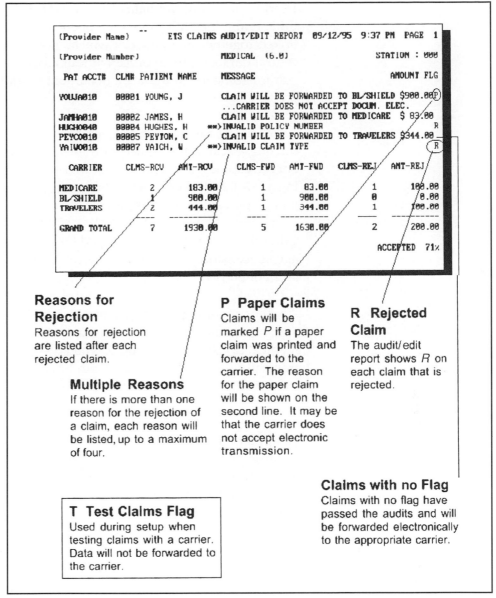

```
(Provider Name)        --    ETS CLAIMS AUDIT/EDIT REPORT  09/12/95  9:37 PM  PAGE  1

(Provider Number)            MEDICAL (6.0)                      STATION : 000

 PAT ACCT#   CLM# PATIENT NAME    MESSAGE                            AMOUNT FLG

YOUJA010    00001 YOUNG, J        CLAIM WILL BE FORWARDED TO BL/SHIELD $900.00 P
                                  ...CARRIER DOES NOT ACCEPT DOCUM. ELEC.
JAMHA010    00002 JAMES, H        CLAIM WILL BE FORWARDED TO MEDICARE  $ 83.00
HUGHO040    00004 HUGHES, H   **>INVALID POLICY NUMBER                        R
PEYCO010    00005 PEYTON, C       CLAIM WILL BE FORWARDED TO TRAVELERS $344.00  R
YAIVO010    00007 YAICH, W    **>INVALID CLAIM TYPE                           R

   CARRIER      CLMS-RCV   AMT-RCV    CLMS-FWD   AMT-FWD   CLMS-REJ   AMT-REJ

 MEDICARE          2        183.00       1        83.00       1       100.00
 BL/SHIELD         1        900.00       1       900.00       0         0.00
 TRAVELERS         2        444.00       1       344.00       1       100.00
                  ---      -------      ---      -------     ---      -------
 GRAND TOTAL       7       1930.00       5      1630.00       2       200.00

                                                            ACCEPTED  71%
```

Reasons for Rejection

Reasons for rejection are listed after each rejected claim.

Multiple Reasons

If there is more than one reason for the rejection of a claim, each reason will be listed, up to a maximum of four.

P Paper Claims

Claims will be marked *P* if a paper claim was printed and forwarded to the carrier. The reason for the paper claim will be shown on the second line. It may be that the carrier does not accept electronic transmission.

R Rejected Claim

The audit/edit report shows *R* on each claim that is rejected.

T Test Claims Flag

Used during setup when testing claims with a carrier. Data will not be forwarded to the carrier.

Claims with no Flag

Claims with no flag have passed the audits and will be forwarded electronically to the appropriate carrier.

Figure 2-4 **Sample audit/edit report.**

e-commerce the exchange of funds over the Internet.

from the standard price, since there is no middleman or distributor in the transaction. These discounts can save the practice a significant amount of money over the course of a year.

ADVANTAGES OF COMPUTERS

In a physician's practice, there are a number of advantages to performing tasks with a computer instead of on paper. First, with a computer database, all the information is located in one place. Pieces of paper and forms are not located in different file cabinets in the office; they are all stored on one computer system.

In addition, computer data can be used by more than one person at a time. If an office has more than one computer, the computers can be linked together in a network which allows them to share files in the central database. In an office without a computer database, it is difficult for someone to update a document if another person is working on it.

Another advantage of computer databases is the simplicity of conducting a search for information. Instead of having to look in different file cabinets and folders, a search can be conducted by just entering a few keystrokes. In a very short time, the information is retrieved and displayed on the computer screen.

Computers also eliminate the need for large amounts of physical storage space, since much of the information is stored in the computer, and not on paper.

Another advantage that computer databases offer over manual filing systems is efficiency. Computers save enormous amounts of time in a medical practice. For example, when medical records are stored electronically, a staff member does not have to pull patient charts at the start of each day and refile them at the end of the day.

From an administrative perspective, the most significant use of the computer in the medical office is to create and process insurance claim forms. When preparing patients' claims, the computer selects information from its databases to create an electronic file of the information needed to complete the claim forms. Those claim forms can then be printed or transmitted electronically.

Bringing computers into the medical office has greatly increased productivity, primarily because computers are much more efficient at processing large amounts of data than human beings. Tasks that would take minutes for a human to complete can be done by the computer in a matter of seconds. For example, suppose a medical practice has multiple providers and hundreds of patients. The phone rings, and a patient would like to know the amount owed on an account. With a computerized billing program in place, the medical office assistant might simply key the first few letters of the patient's last name into the computer, causing the patient's account to appear on the screen. The outstanding balance then could be communicated to the patient.

In another example, suppose the wrong diagnosis code has been written on an insurance claim form, and the claim has been rejected by the insurance carrier. To resubmit the claim without the use of a computer might require the entire form to be completed again by hand. However, if the medical office used a computerized billing program, the error could be corrected in seconds and a new form either printed or submitted electronically.

Computers not only make the medical office more efficient, they also reduce errors. Working with a computer system, information is entered once and then used over and over again. Provided the information is entered correctly the first time, it will be correct every time it is used. For example, information such as the patient's address and insurance policy number is entered in the computer once. The computer stores the information, and when the information is needed to fill out a claim form, the computer locates it and uses it to complete the task, such as printing a completed claim form. The next time a claim needs to be created, the computer goes through the same process, using the same information. Without a computer, someone would have to key all the information on an insurance form each time a claim was being submitted for the patient. Not only does this consume more time, but it introduces the possibility of error every time the information has to be rekeyed.

Computerized billing systems also make it easier to focus on checking that procedure and diagnosis codes are related in the correct way. This is essential if insurance claims are to be paid in a timely manner. If a procedure code does not relate to the diagnosis code, the claim will be rejected, even though the procedure may be one that is covered under the patient's policy. For example, suppose a patient saw the doctor and was diagnosed with acute sinusitis. The physician ordered X rays of the patient's sinus cavities in order to arrive at this diagnosis. However, the procedure code was incorrectly entered as a forearm X ray. The insurance company will not pay the claim because the procedure is not related to the diagnosis.

While computers do increase the efficiency of the medical office and reduce errors, they are not more accurate than the individual entering the data. If human errors occur while entering the information, the data coming out of the computer will be incorrect. Computers are very precise and also very unforgiving. While the human brain knows that flu is short for influenza, the computer does not know this, and it regards them as two distinct conditions. If a computer operator accidentally enters a name as "ORourke" instead of "O'Rourke," a human might know what is meant; the computer does not. It would probably respond with a message such as "No such patient exists in the database."

Most human errors occur during data entry, such as pressing the wrong key on the keyboard, or because of the lack of computer literacy—not knowing how to use a program to accomplish the tasks. For this reason, proper training in data-entry techniques and the use of computer programs are essential for medical office personnel who are working with computers.

CHAPTER REVIEW

USING TERMINOLOGY

Match the terms on the left with the definitions on the right.

_____ 1. audit/edit report

_____ 2. clearinghouse

_____ 3. database

_____ 4. e-commerce

_____ 5. electronic funds transfer (EFT)

_____ 6. electronic media claim (EMC)

_____ 7. electronic medical records (EMR)

_____ 8. health informatics

_____ 9. walkout receipt

a. The electronic collection and management of health data.

b. An insurance claim that is sent by a computer over a telephone line using a modem.

c. A system that transfers money electronically from one account to another.

d. Information about patients, such as medical history, lab results, and so on, that is stored on a computer rather than paper.

e. The exchange of funds over the Internet.

f. A service bureau that collects electronic insurance claims and forwards them to the appropriate insurance carriers.

g. A report from a clearinghouse that lists errors that need to be corrected before a claim can be submitted to the insurance carrier.

h. A document listing charges and payments that is given to a patient after an office visit.

i. A collection of related facts.

CHECKING YOUR UNDERSTANDING

Write "T" or "F" in the blank to indicate whether you think the statement is true or false.

_____ 10. One method of increasing the security of medical data stored on a computer is to assign passwords to all users.

_____ 11. Computerized scheduling makes it easier to reschedule appointments in a medical office.

_____ 12. Online databases store personal information on patient diagnoses.

_____ 13. Most states do not have laws that protect the privacy of a patient's medical records.

_____ **14.** Electronic media claims are usually paid in about the same number of days as claims submitted on paper forms.

_____ **15.** Clearinghouses perform audits of claim data before transmitting them to insurance carriers.

Answer the questions below in the space provided.

16. List two advantages of using computers in the medical office.

_____

_____

17. Explain the advantage of electronic medical records over traditional paper records in an emergency situation.

_____

_____

Choose the best answer.

_____ **18.** Electronic remittance advice (ERA) is:
   a. the electronic transfer of funds from one bank account to another
   b. a report from a clearinghouse listing any errors in a claim
   c. an electronic explanation of benefits

_____ **19.** Systems that allow physicians' clinical notes to be stored in a computer are known as:
   a. Internet applications
   b. electronic medical records applications
   c. diagnosis coding applications

_____ **20.** E-commerce allows medical practices to:
   a. track changes in computer data by individual user
   b. purchase supplies over the Internet
   c. safeguard confidential patient medical records that are stored on a computer.

MediSoft for Windows Training

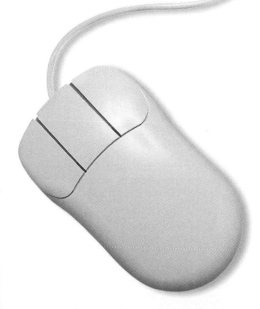

3 Introduction to MediSoft

WHAT YOU NEED TO KNOW

To use this chapter, you need to know how to:
- Start your computer and Microsoft Windows 98.
- Use the keyboard and mouse.

OBJECTIVES

In this chapter, you will learn how to:
- Start MediSoft.
- Use the Student Data Disk.
- Move around the MediSoft menus.
- Use the MediSoft toolbar.
- Enter, edit, and delete data in MediSoft.
- Save and back up MediSoft data.
- Use MediSoft's Help features.
- Exit MediSoft.

KEY TERMS

backup data   MMDDCCYY format
balloon help   transactions
knowledge base

WHAT IS MEDISOFT?

MediSoft is a patient accounting software program. Information on patients, providers, insurance carriers, and patient and insurance billing is stored and processed by the system. MediSoft is widely used by medical practices throughout the United States. It is typically used to accomplish the following daily work in a medical practice:

◆ Enter information on new patients, and change information on established patients as needed.

◆ Enter transactions, such as charges, to patients' accounts.

◆ Record payments and adjustments from patients and insurance companies.

◆ Print walkout receipts and statements for patients.

◆ Submit insurance claims to carriers.

◆ Print standard reports, and create custom reports.

◆ Schedule appointments.

Many of the general working concepts used in operating MediSoft are similar to those in other software programs. Thus, you should be able to transfer many skills taught in this book to other patient accounting programs.

HOW MEDISOFT DATA IS ORGANIZED AND STORED

Information entered into MediSoft is stored in databases. As defined in Chapter 2, a database is a collection of related pieces of information.

MEDISOFT DATABASES MediSoft stores these major types of data:

◆ **Provider Data** The provider database has information about the physician(s) as well as the practice, such as its name and address, phone number, and tax and medical identifier numbers.

◆ **Patient Data** Each patient information form is stored in the patient database. The patient's unique chart number and personal information—name and address, phone number, birth date, Social Security number, gender, marital status, and employer—are examples of information stored in this database.

◆ **Insurance Carriers** The insurance carrier database contains the names, addresses, and other data about each insurance carrier used by patients, such as the type of plan. Usually, this database also contains information on each carrier's electronic media claim (EMC) submission.

- **Diagnosis Codes** The diagnosis code database contains the *International Classification of Diseases, 9th Revision, Clinical Modification (ICD-9)* codes that indicate the reason a service is provided. The codes entered in this database are those most frequently used by the practice. The practice's superbill often serves as a source document when the MediSoft system is first set up.

- **Procedure Codes** The procedure code database contains the data needed to create charges. The *Current Procedural Terminology (CPT)* codes most often used by the practice are selected for this database. The practice's superbill is often a good source document for these codes. Other claim data elements, such as place of service (POS) and the charge for each procedure, are also stored in the procedure code database.

- **Transactions** The transaction database stores information about each patient's visits, diagnoses, and procedures, as well as received and outstanding payments. **Transactions** in the form of charges, payments, and adjustments are also stored in the transaction database.

transactions *charges, payments, and adjustments.*

Within MediSoft, each database is linked, or related, to each of the others by having at least one fact in common. For example, information entered in the patient database is shared with the transaction database, linking the two. Information is entered only once; MediSoft selects the data from each database as needed.

USING THE STUDENT DATA DISK

Before a medical office begins using MediSoft, basic information about the practice and its patients must be entered in the computer. For the exercises you will complete in this book, the preliminary work has been done for you. The MediSoft databases for these exercises are stored on the Student Data Disk located inside the back cover.

The Student Data Disk contains a folder that includes the data for the practice used in this book, the Family Care Center (FCC). Before you begin using the Student Data Disk, you need to make a working copy of it, following the instructions below. When you are finished making the disk copy, store the original Student Data Disk in a safe place. You may need to use it to make another copy if the working disk is accidentally damaged or lost.

Complete the following steps to make a copy of the Student Data Disk. If your computer has a version of Windows other than Windows 98, ask your instructor for alternate directions.

1. Turn on the computer and monitor.

2. After the Windows 98 desktop is displayed, insert the Student Data Disk in the 3½" floppy drive (drive A).

3. Double-click the My Computer icon on the desktop. The My Computer window is displayed.

4. Click the icon labeled "3½ Floppy (A:)."

5. On the File menu, click Copy Disk. The Copy Disk dialog box is displayed.

6. The Copy From and Copy To windows should both have "3½ Floppy (A:)" highlighted. If they are not highlighted, click 3½ Floppy (A:) in both the Copy From and Copy To windows.

7. Click the Start button. The computer begins reading the files on the source disk. You can monitor the computer's progress by viewing the bar above the words "Reading source disk."

8. When the system prompts you to insert the disk you want to copy to (the destination disk), eject the Student Data Disk from the drive.

9. Insert a blank disk in the floppy drive, and click the OK button. The files are copied to the destination disk. Again, you can monitor the progress by looking at the bar above the words "Writing to destination disk."

10. When the copy is completed, the message "Copy completed successfully" is displayed. Eject the disk from the drive, and label it "Working Copy FCC."

11. Close the Copy Disk dialog box by clicking the Close button.

12. Close the My Computer dialog box by clicking the Close button (in this case, the X in the upper right corner).

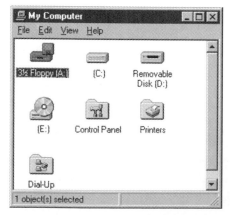

Sample My Computer window with 3½ Floppy (A:) icon highlighted.

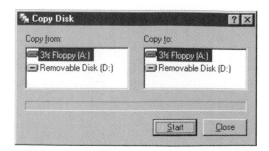

Copy Disk dialog box.

STARTING MEDISOFT

To begin using MediSoft, it is necessary to have a basic understanding of how to start the program; enter, edit, and save data; and exit the program. This section provides that information.

The following exercise describes how to start the MediSoft program for the first time.

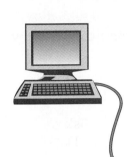

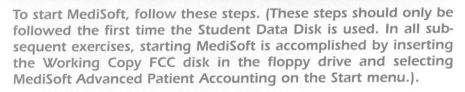
Exercise 3-1

To start MediSoft, follow these steps. (These steps should only be followed the first time the Student Data Disk is used. In all subsequent exercises, starting MediSoft is accomplished by inserting the Working Copy FCC disk in the floppy drive and selecting MediSoft Advanced Patient Accounting on the Start menu.).

1. Insert the Working Copy FCC disk in the floppy drive (This is usually the A: drive; if your computer uses a different letter to represent the floppy drive, please substitute that letter for "A:" whenever it appears in these instructions.)

2. While holding down the F7 key, click Start, Programs, MediSoft, MediSoft Advanced Patient Accounting to start MediSoft. When the Find MediSoft Database dialog box appears, release the F7 key. This dialog box asks you to enter the MediSoft data directory.

3. Click the bar that reads "Find MediSoft Database" at the top of the dialog box to make the dialog box active. (If you do not click on the dialog box before keying, your keystrokes will not appear in the white box.) Then key *A:\MEDIDATA* in the space provided. The dialog box should now look like this:

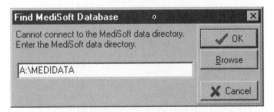

4. Click the OK button. The Create Data dialog box is displayed.

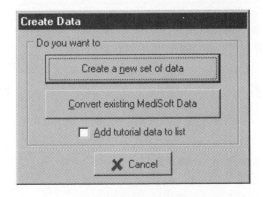

5. Click the Create a New Set of Data button. The Create a New Set of Data dialog box appears. In the upper box, key *Family Care Center*. In the lower box, key *FCC*. The dialog box should now look like this:

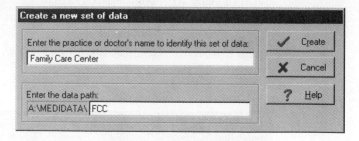

6. Click the Create button. A Warning dialog box is displayed.

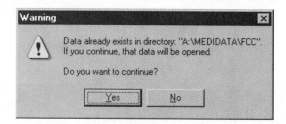

7. Click the Yes button. The Practice Information box appears.

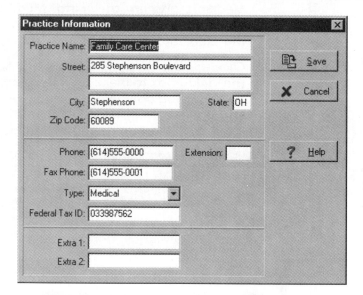

8. Click the Save button. The Family Care Center practice is open. Your screen should look like the one pictured on page 43.

9. To exit MediSoft, click Exit on the File menu.

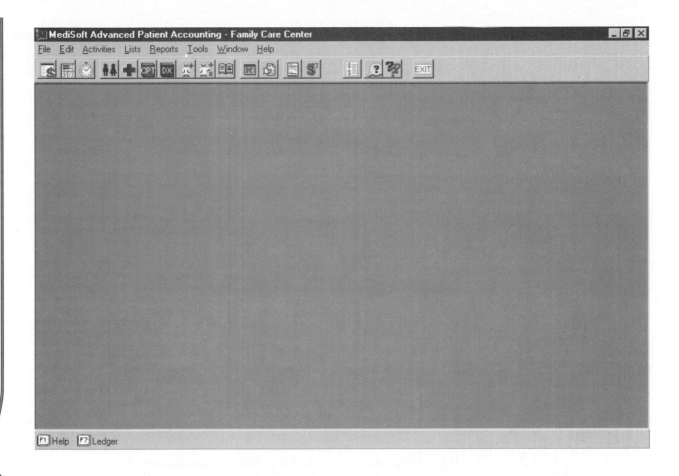

Any time you want to enter MediSoft to work on exercises, be sure you insert the Working Copy FCC disk in drive A: before you start the MediSoft program.

THE MEDISOFT MENU BAR

MediSoft offers choices of actions through a series of menus. Commands are issued by clicking an option on the menu bar or by clicking a shortcut button on the toolbar. The menu bar lists the names of the menus in MediSoft: File, Edit, Activities, Lists, Reports, Tools, Window, and Help (see Figure 3-1 on page 44). Beneath each menu name is a pull-down menu of one or more options.

File Menu   The File menu is used to enter information about the medical office practice when first setting up MediSoft. It is also used to back up data, restore data, set program security options, and change the program date (see Figure 3-2 on page 44).

Edit Menu   The Edit menu contains the basic commands needed to move, change, or delete information (see Figure 3-3 on page 44). These commands are Cut, Copy, Paste, and Delete.

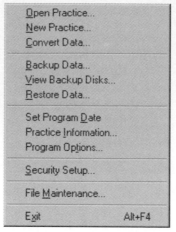

Figure 3-2
File menu.

Figure 3-3
Edit menu.

Activities Menu   Most medical office data collected on a day-to-day basis are entered through options on the Activities menu (see Figure 3-4). This menu is used to enter financial transactions, create insurance claims, view summaries of patient account information, calculate billing charges, and access Office Hours, MediSoft's built-in appointment scheduler. Transactions include charges, payments, and adjustments.

Lists Menu   Information on new patients, such as name, address, and employer, is entered through the Lists menu (see Figure 3-5). If information needs to be changed on an established patient, it is also updated through this menu. The Lists menu also provides access to lists of codes, insurance carriers, and providers. These lists may be updated and printed when necessary.

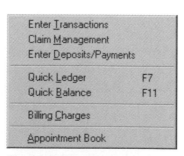

Figure 3-4
Activities menu.

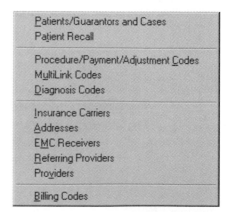

Figure 3-5
Lists menu.

Reports Menu The Reports menu is used to print reports about patients' accounts and other reports about the practice (see Figure 3-6). MediSoft comes with a number of standard report formats, such as day sheets, aging reports, and patient ledgers. Practices may create their own report formats using the Design Custom Reports and Bills option.

Tools Menu The built-in calculator is accessed through the Tools menu. Other options on the Tools menu can be used to view the contents of a file as well as a profile of the computer system (see Figure 3-7).

Window Menu Using the Window menu, it is possible to switch back and forth between several open windows. For example, if the Transaction Entry dialog box and the Patient List dialog box were both open, the Window menu would look like the menu in Figure 3-8. The Window menu also has an option to close all windows.

SHORT CUT The easiest way to switch back and forth between two or more open windows is to click anywhere on a window to make it the active window. Clicking on a window makes it active and automatically deselects the previously active window.

Help Menu The Help menu, shown in Figure 3-9, is used to access MediSoft's built-in Help feature and also provides a link to MediSoft support on the World Wide Web.

Exercise 3-2

Practice using the MediSoft menus.

1. **Start MediSoft.**

2. **Click the Lists menu on the menu bar.**

3. **Click Patients/Guarantors and Cases. The Patient List dialog box is displayed (see Figure 3-10 on page 46).**

4. **Click the Close button at the bottom of the dialog box.**

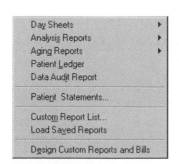

Day Sheets ▶
Analysis Reports ▶
Aging Reports ▶
Patient Ledger
Data Audit Report

Patient Statements...

Custom Report List...
Load Saved Reports

Design Custom Reports and Bills

Figure 3-6
Reports menu.

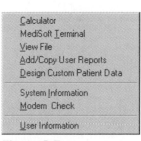

Calculator
MediSoft Terminal
View File
Add/Copy User Reports
Design Custom Patient Data

System Information
Modem Check

User Information

Figure 3-7
Tools menu.

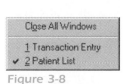

Close All Windows

1 Transaction Entry
✔ 2 Patient List

Figure 3-8
Window menu.

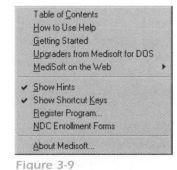

Table of Contents
How to Use Help
Getting Started
Upgraders from Medisoft for DOS
MediSoft on the Web ▶

✔ Show Hints
✔ Show Shortcut Keys
Register Program...
NDC Enrollment Forms

About Medisoft...

Figure 3-9
Help menu.

5. Click the Activities menu.

6. Click Enter Transactions. The Transaction Entry dialog box is displayed (see Figure 3-11).

7. Click the Close button.

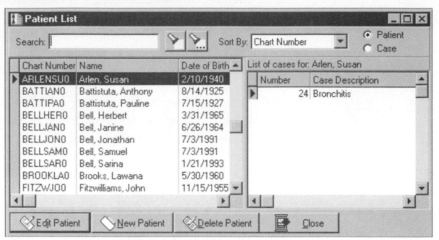

Figure 3-10 **Patient List dialog box.**

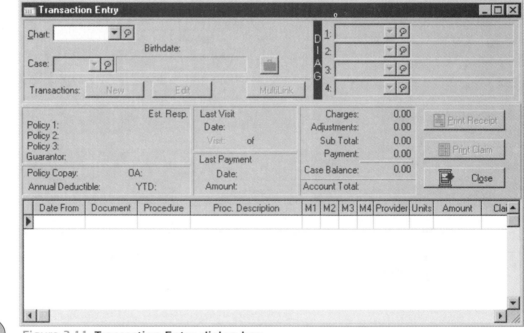

Figure 3-11 **Transaction Entry dialog box.**

THE MEDISOFT TOOLBAR

Located below the menu bar, the toolbar contains a series of buttons with icons that represent the most common activities performed in MediSoft. These buttons are shortcuts for frequently used menu commands. The toolbar displays 18 buttons (see Figure 3-12 and Table 3-1).

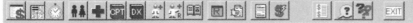

Figure 3-12 **MediSoft toolbar.**

Table 3-1   Toolbar Buttons

Button	Button Name	Associated Function	Activity
	Transaction Entry	Transaction Entry dialog box	Enter transactions.
	Claim Management	Claim Management dialog box	Create and send insurance claims.
	Appointment Book	Office Hours	Schedule appointments.
	Patient List	Patient List dialog box	Enter and edit patient information.
	Insurance Carrier List	Insurance Carrier List dialog box	Add, edit, or delete insurance carriers.
	Procedure Code List	Procedure/Payment/Adjustment List dialog box	Add, edit, or delete procedure, payment, and adjustment codes.
	Diagnosis Code List	Diagnosis List dialog box	Add, edit, or delete diagnosis codes.
	Provider List	Provider List dialog box	Add, edit, or delete providers.
	Referring Provider List	Referring Provider List dialog box	Add, edit, or delete referring providers.
	Address List	Address List dialog box	Add, edit, or delete addresses.
	Patient Recall Entry	Patient Recall dialog box	Add a patient to the recall list.
	Custom Report List	Open Report dialog box	Display or print reports.
	Quick Ledger	Quick Ledger dialog box	View data in patient ledger.
	Quick Balance	Quick Balance dialog box	View patient account balance.
	Deposit/Payment Entry	Deposit List	Enter deposits and payments.
	Show/Hide Hints	Balloon help	Turn the Hints feature on or off.
	Help	Contents dialog box	Access MediSoft's online help files.
	Exit the MediSoft Program	Exit	Exit the MediSoft program.

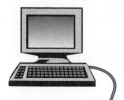

Exercise 3-3

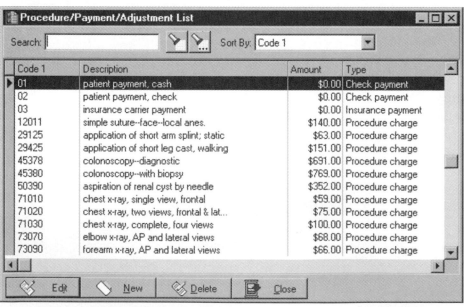

Practice using buttons on the toolbar.

1. Click the Provider List button. The Provider List dialog box is displayed (see Figure 3-13).

2. Click the Close button to close the dialog box.

3. Click the Procedure Code List button. The Procedure/Payment/ Adjustment List dialog box is displayed (see Figure 3-14).

4. Click the Close button to close the dialog box.

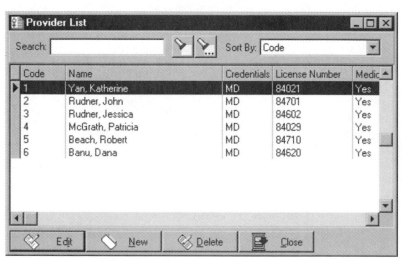

Figure 3-13 **Provider List dialog box.**

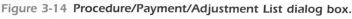

Figure 3-14 **Procedure/Payment/Adjustment List dialog box.**

ENTERING AND EDITING DATA

All data, whether patients' addresses or charges for procedures, are entered into MediSoft through the menus on the menu bar or through the buttons on the toolbar. Selecting an option from the menus or toolbar brings up a dialog box. The Tab key is used to move between text boxes within a dialog box. In some dialog boxes, information is entered by keying data into a text box. For example, a patient's name would be keyed directly into a text box. At other times selections are made from a list of choices already present. For example, when entering the name of the provider a patient is seeing, the provider is selected from a drop-down list of providers already in the system.

SHORT CUT To make a selection from a drop-down list, either of these techniques can be used: the scroll bars can be used to scroll up or down the list until the desired entry is displayed, or, the first few letters of the desired entry can be keyed in the text box next to the drop-down list. When characters are keyed, the system displays the entry in the list that most closely matches the characters keyed. When the desired entry appears highlighted, the Enter key is pressed. In most instances, the latter method is much quicker than using the scroll bars to locate the desired entry. Imagine a practice with 3000 patients. To locate a patient named Zawacki using the scroll method would require scrolling down a very long list. Keying in the first few letters of the patient's chart number, in this case "ZAW," would cause the system to display the first entry beginning with those letters. (Chart numbers are discussed in Chapter 4.)

DATES MediSoft is a date-sensitive program. When transactions are entered in the program, the dates must be accurate, or the data entered will be of little value to the practice. Many times, date-sensitive information is not entered into MediSoft on the same day that the event or transaction occurred. For example, Friday afternoon's office visits may not be entered into the program until Monday. If the MediSoft Program Date is not changed to Friday's date before entering the data, all the information entered on Monday will be stored as Monday's transactions. For this reason, it is important to know how to change the MediSoft Program Date.

For most of the exercises in this book, you will need to change the MediSoft Program Date to the date specified at the beginning of the exercise. The following steps are used to change the MediSoft Program Date:

1. Click Set Program Date on the File menu, or click the date displayed on the status bar. A pop-up calendar is displayed.

2. Click the desired month in the Month drop-down list.

3. Select the desired year by clicking the counter button next to the year.

4. Select the desired date by clicking on that date in the calendar.

5. To save the changes, press Enter or click the green Checkmark button just to the left of the month field.

6. To exit the pop-up calendar without saving the date change, click the red Cancel button.

MMDDCCYY format *a specific way in which dates must be keyed, in which "MM" stands for month, "DD" stands for day, "CC" stands for century, and "YY" stands for year.*

In most MediSoft dialog boxes, dates are entered in the MMDDCCYY format. The **MMDDCCYY format** is a specific way in which dates must be keyed. "MM" stands for the month, "DD" stands for the day, "CC" represents century, and "YY" stands for the year. Each day, month, century, and year entry must contain two digits, and no punctuation can be used. For example, the date of February 1, 2004, would be keyed as "02012004."

Figure 3-15 **Pop-up Calendar button.**

SHORT CUT In most MediSoft dialog boxes, dates can be keyed in the text boxes or selected from a pop-up calendar. When the Pop-up Calendar button (see Figure 3-15) is clicked inside a dialog box, a small calendar appears on the screen. You can use this small calendar to change the date, as described above.

Exercise 3-4

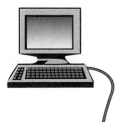

Practice entering information and correcting errors.

Date: November 1, 2004

1. **Click the Activities menu.**

2. **Click Enter Transactions.**

3. **Click the triangle button in the Chart box. The Chart drop-down list is displayed (see Figure 3-16).**

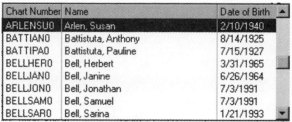

Figure 3-16 **Chart drop-down list.**

4. To select James Smith, key the first two letters of his chart number (SMITHJAØ): *SM*

   Notice that when "SM" was keyed, the system went to the entry for the first patient whose chart number begins with "SM," in this case James Smith.

5. Press the Enter key.

6. Click the Edit button. The Charge tab is displayed (see Figure 3-17 on page 52).

7. Click the Pop-up Calendar button that is next to the first Dates box. Click November in the drop-down list and click 7 in the calendar to change the day to November 7. To save the date change, click the button to the left of the month entry that contains a green check mark.

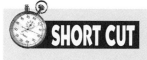 To save the date change, you can press the Enter key instead of clicking the green checkmark.

8. Click the second Dates text box. Notice that the system automatically changes the entry to match the date in the first Dates box. Press the Enter key to close the calendar.

9. Look at the Amount box, where "142.00" is displayed.

10. Click the Procedure box. Then key *99203*. The system highlights the procedure in the drop-down list.

11. Press the Enter key.

12. Look at the Amount box again. The charge associated with the new procedure code, "120.00," is displayed (see Figure 3-17 on page 52). The system automatically changes the entry in the amount field to match the entry in the Procedure field.

13. Change the entry in the Amount box from 120.00 to 125.00 by highlighting 120.00, keying *125*, and pressing the Enter key. The amount displayed changes to 125.00. Notice how the system automatically adds the decimal point.

Pop-up Calendar buttons

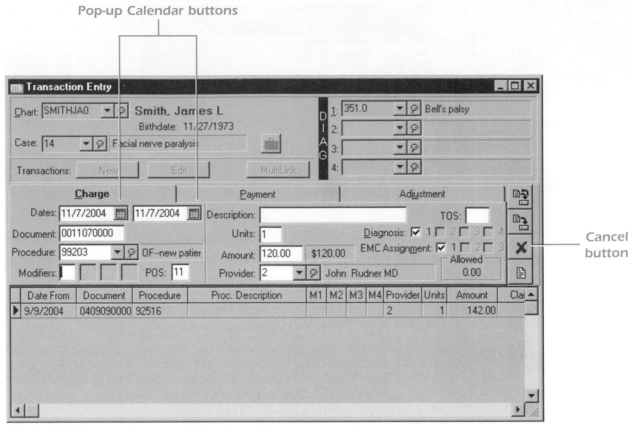

Cancel button

Figure 3-17 Transaction Entry dialog box with data entered.

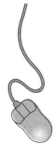

14. Press the Tab key repeatedly and watch as the cursor moves from box to box.

15. Exit the Transaction Entry dialog box without saving these changes. To do this, click the Cancel button at the right side of the dialog box that displays a red "X."

16. You are now back at the main Transaction Entry dialog box. To close this dialog box, click the Close button.

SAVING DATA

Information entered into MediSoft is saved by clicking the Save button that appears in most dialog boxes (those in which data have been input). In an office setting, data are saved to the computer's hard drive. In this book, however, all data must be saved to the Working Copy disk in drive A. This allows each student working with MediSoft to complete the exercises in the book independently. If one student saved data to the hard drive, the next student would find the data already in the system when attempting to complete the exercises.

DELETING DATA

In some MediSoft dialog boxes, there are buttons for the purpose of deleting data. For example, to delete an insurance carrier, the entry for the carrier is clicked in the Insurance Carrier List dialog box. Then, the Delete button is clicked. MediSoft will ask for a confirmation before deleting the data. In other dialog boxes, such as the Transaction Entry dialog box, there is no button for deleting data. In this situation, the method for deleting data is less obvious. The entry to be deleted is clicked, and then the right mouse button is clicked. A shortcut menu is displayed that contains an option to delete the transaction. Again, MediSoft will ask for confirmation before deleting the data.

BACKING UP DATA

backup data *a copy of data files at a specific point in time that can be used to restore data to the system.*

Data is periodically saved on removable magnetic media, such as diskettes or tapes, through a process known as backing up. **Backup data** is a copy of data files made at a specific point in time that can be used to restore data to the system. Backups are performed on a regular schedule, determined by the medical practice. Many practices back up data at the end of each day. Backups are only for an office setting. In this book, the steps required to back up data will be covered, but an actual backup will not be performed.

USING MEDISOFT HELP

MediSoft offers users three different types of help.

balloon help *information provided through a series of balloons that appear on the screen.*

Balloon Help Balloon help is information provided through a series of balloons that appear on the screen as the mouse pointer is moved to certain items. The balloons contain text that explains the purpose of the particular item (see Figure 3-18). The text in the balloon also appears on the status bar at the bottom of the screen.

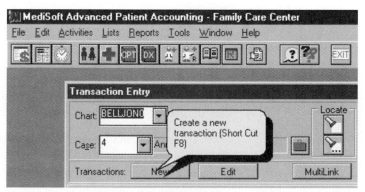

Figure 3-18 *Example of balloon help.*

Built-in Help For more detailed help, MediSoft has an extensive help feature built into the program itself, which is accessed through the Help menu.

Online Help The Help menu also provides access to MediSoft help available on the MediSoft corporate Web site, www.medisoft.com. The Web site contains a searchable **knowledge base**, which is a collection of up-to-date technical information about all MediSoft products.

knowledge base *a collection of up-to-date technical information.*

Exercise 3-5

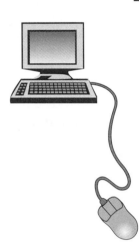

Practice using MediSoft's built-in help feature.

1. Click the Help menu.

2. Click Table of Contents. MediSoft displays a list of topics for which help is available.

3. Click Diagnosis Entry. Information on entering diagnosis codes is displayed.

4. Print the information by clicking the Print button. The Print dialog box is displayed.

5. Click the OK button to print.

6. To exit Help, click File on the Help menu bar. Then click Exit.

Exercise 3-6 .

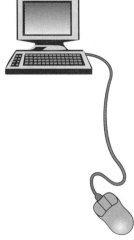

Practice using MediSoft's online help.

1. Access the World Wide Web.

2. Go to MediSoft's Web site, www.medisoft.com

3. Click the underlined link to the knowledge base.

4. Click the option to perform a keyword search.

5. Key *payments* in the Search box.

6. Click the Search button.

7. Review the results of the search.

8. Terminate your Internet connection, if appropriate.

9. Click the Exit button on the toolbar to exit MediSoft.

EXITING MEDISOFT

MediSoft is exited by clicking Exit on the File menu or by clicking the Exit button on the toolbar. To avoid the inconvenience of exiting and restarting MediSoft many times during a day when the computer is needed for a different program, MediSoft can be made temporarily inactive by using the Minimize button, the first of the three small buttons displayed in the upper-right corner of the window. MediSoft can be reactivated at any time by clicking the MediSoft button on the Windows 98 taskbar (see Figure 3-19).

Figure 3-19 **Sample Windows taskbar with MediSoft button.**

CHAPTER REVIEW

USING TERMINOLOGY

Match the terms on the left with the definitions on the right.

_____ **1.** backup data

_____ **2.** balloon help

_____ **3.** knowledge base

_____ **4.** MMDDCCYY format

_____ **5.** transactions

a. Help provided through a series of balloons that appear on the screen as the cursor moves to certain items.

b. A searchable collection of up-to-date technical information.

c. In MediSoft, charges, payments, and adjustments.

d. A way in which dates must be keyed.

e. A copy of data files made at a specific point in time that can be used to restore data to the system.

CHECKING YOUR UNDERSTANDING

Answer the questions below in the space provided.

6. Describe two ways of issuing a command in MediSoft.

_____

_____

7. What are two ways data are entered in a box?

_____

_____

8. What three types of MediSoft help are available?

_____

_____

_____

9. Which menu provides access to Office Hours, MediSoft's scheduling feature?

_____

10. What is the purpose of the buttons on the toolbar?

_____

_____

11. What is the format for entering dates in MediSoft?

_____

12. Describe two ways of exiting MediSoft.

_____

_____

APPLYING KNOWLEDGE

13. Use MediSoft's Built-in Help to look up information on the following topics:

   • How to enter diagnosis codes

   • How to print procedure code lists from the MediSoft database

AT THE COMPUTER

Answer the following questions at the computer:

14. How many options are there in the Reports menu?

_____

15. What is the first choice on the Lists menu?

_____

16. List the options on the Activities menu.

_____

17. Set the MediSoft Program Date to December 1, 2004, and then exit MediSoft.

Entering Patient Information

WHAT YOU NEED TO KNOW

To use this chapter, you need to know how to:

◆ Start MediSoft.

◆ Move around the MediSoft menus.

◆ Use the MediSoft toolbar.

◆ Enter and edit data in MediSoft.

◆ Exit MediSoft.

OBJECTIVES

In this chapter, you will learn how to:

◆ Use the MediSoft Search feature.

◆ Assign a chart number for a new patient.

◆ Enter personal and employer information for a new patient.

◆ Locate and change information for an established patient.

KEY TERMS

chart number
guarantor

HOW PATIENT INFORMATION IS ORGANIZED IN MEDISOFT

Figure 4-1
**Patient List
shortcut button.**

Patient information is accessed through the Patient List dialog box. The Patient List dialog box is displayed when Patients/Guarantors and Cases is clicked on the Lists menu or when the corresponding shortcut button is clicked on the toolbar (see Figure 4-1).

The Patient List dialog box (see Figure 4-2) is divided into two primary sections. The left side of the window displays information about patients, and the right side of the window contains information about cases. Cases are covered in Chapter 5. At the top right side of the Patient List dialog box, there are two radio buttons: Patient and Case. When the Patient radio button is clicked, the left side of the window becomes active. Correspondingly, when the Case radio button is clicked, the right side of the window becomes active. The command buttons at the bottom of the dialog box vary, depending on which side of the window is active.

The Patient window contains the following data: Chart Number, Name, Date of Birth, Social Security Number, Patient ID #2, Patient Type, Phone 1, Provider, Last Name, Billing Code, and Patient Indicator. There is not enough room in the Patient window to display all this information, so only a portion is visible at one time. To view the rest of the patient information, it is necessary to use the scroll bars. Scrolling to the right displays information in the additional columns, including Social Security Number, Patient ID #2, and so on. Scrolling down the Patient window displays additional chart numbers and patient names (see Figure 4-3). The command buttons at the bottom of the screen include: Edit Patient, New Patient, Delete Patient, and Close.

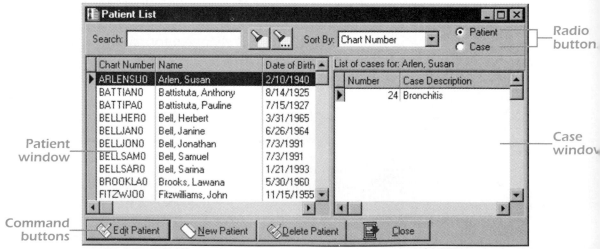

Figure 4-2 **Patient List dialog box.**

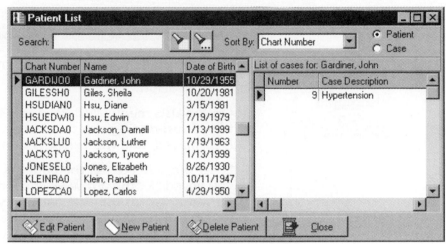

Figure 4-3 **Patient List dialog box with scroll bars in use.**

SEARCHING FOR PATIENT INFORMATION

A patient who comes to a medical practice for the first time fills out a patient information form. The information on this form needs to be entered into the MediSoft patient/guarantor database before any insurance claims can be submitted. However, before information on a patient is entered into the system, it is important to search the database to be certain that the patient does not already exist in the database.

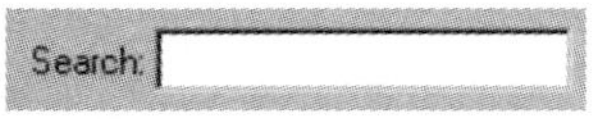

Search:

Figure 4-4 **Search box.**

MediSoft's Search feature is used to look for information on patients, insurance carriers, diagnosis codes, and procedure codes, as well as the names and addresses of employers and providers. Searches for information on patients are conducted using the Search box in the upper left corner of the Patient List dialog box (see Figure 4-4).

In a search, MediSoft locates the name or number that most closely matches the letters and/or numbers entered in the Search box. For example, if the letters "SMI" are entered in the Search box, MediSoft will match the first patient with a last name beginning with the letters "SMI." The Search box for patients can contain up to seven letters, including spaces.

TIP> It does not matter whether capital letters or lowercase letters are entered in the Search box. For example, keying "SMITH," "Smith," or "smith" will all locate the first patient in the database with the last name of Smith.

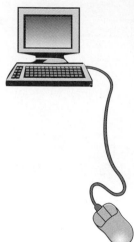

Exercise 4-1

Use the Search feature to locate information on James Smolowski.

1. **Start MediSoft.**

2. **On the Lists menu, click Patients/Guarantors and Cases or click the corresponding shortcut button. The Patient List dialog box is displayed, and the cursor is blinking in the Search box.**

3. **Enter the first letter of the patient's last name. Notice that when you keyed "S," the arrow on the left side of the Patient window moved down to the first patient whose name begins with the letter "S," Jill Simmons. Continue entering the patient's last name. As soon as you key the next two letters, "mo," the arrow points to James Smolowski. Smolowski is the only patient whose name begins with the letters "Smo."**

4. **Click the Close button to exit the Patient List dialog box.**

ENTERING NEW PATIENT INFORMATION

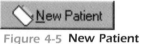

Figure 4-5 **New Patient button.**

Information on a new patient is entered in MediSoft by clicking the New Patient button at the bottom of the Patient List dialog box (see Figure 4-5). This action opens the Patient/Guarantor dialog box (see Figure 4-6). The Patient/Guarantor dialog box contains two tabs: the Name, Address tab and the Other Information tab.

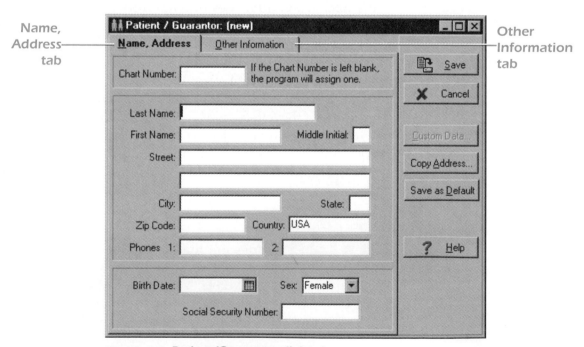

Figure 4-6 **Patient/Guarantor dialog box.**

NAME, ADDRESS TAB

The Name, Address tab is where basic patient information is entered.

Chart Number

chart number *a unique number that identifies a patient.*

The **chart number** is a unique number that identifies a patient. In MediSoft, a chart number links together all the information about a patient that is stored in the different databases, such as name, address, charges, insurance claims, and so on. Each patient is assigned an eight-character chart number. If the chart number box for a patient is left blank, the system will assign a chart number.

Medical practices may use different methods for assigning chart numbers, although these general guidelines must be followed:

- The chart number must start with a letter but can contain a combination of letters and numbers.

- No special characters, such as hyphens, periods, or spaces, are allowed.

- No two chart numbers can be the same.

For the purposes of this book, the following method will be used for assigning chart numbers:

- The first five characters of the chart number are the first five letters of a patient's last name. If the patient's last name is less than five characters, add the beginning letters of the patient's first name.

- The next two characters are usually the first two letters of a patient's first name. (If the first two letters of the first name were used to complete the first five letters, the next two letters of the patient's first name are used.)

- The last character is always a zero, displayed in this book with the symbol "Ø."

For example, the chart number for John Fitzwilliams would begin with the first five letters of his last name (FITZW), followed by the first two characters of his first name (JO), followed by a zero (Ø). John's complete chart number would be FITZWJOØ. Following the same rules, John's daughter Sarah would have a chart number of FITZWSAØ.

Exercise 4-2

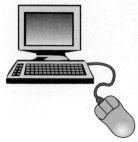

Create a chart number for each of these patients.

Albert Wong _____

Jessica Sypkowski _____

John James_____

Personal Data

In addition to the chart number, personal information about a patient is entered in the Name, Address tab.

Name, Address, and Phone Numbers The boxes for name, address, and phone numbers contain basic information about a patient. There are two boxes for phones: the one on the left (1) is for the phone number; the one on the right (2) is for the fax number. If there is no fax number, this box is left blank or an alternate phone number is listed. Phone numbers and fax numbers must be entered without parentheses or hyphens.

Birth Date The patient's birth date is entered in the Birth Date box using the MMDDCCYY format.

Sex This drop-down list contains choices for the patient's gender, male or female.

Social Security Number The nine-digit Social Security number should be entered with hyphens; however, the system will accept the number if entered without them.

OTHER INFORMATION TAB

The Other Information tab within the Patient/Guarantor dialog box contains facts about a patient's employment and other miscellaneous information (see Figure 4-7).

Type The Type drop-down list is used to designate whether, for billing purposes, an individual is a patient or guarantor (see Figure 4-8).

In the MediSoft Patient/Guarantor dialog box, individuals are classified into two categories: patient and guarantor. *Patient* is used to refer to individuals who are patients of the practice, whether or not they are also the insurance policyholder. The term **guarantor** refers to an individual who is not a patient of the practice, but who is the insurance policyholder for a patient of the practice. For example, a parent

guarantor *an individual who is a policyholder for a patient of the practice.*

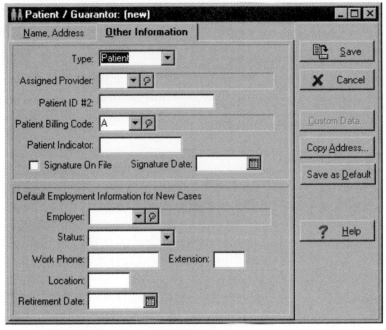

Figure 4-7 **Other Information tab.**

may not be a patient of the practice, but may be the individual whose insurance policy provides coverage for a child who is a patient. In this case, the child is the patient and the parent is the guarantor.

Information about the patient is always entered in MediSoft in the Name/Address tab. When the patient is not the policyholder, information about the guarantor must also be entered in the MediSoft database for insurance claims to be processed. This information is collected from the patient information or patient update form.

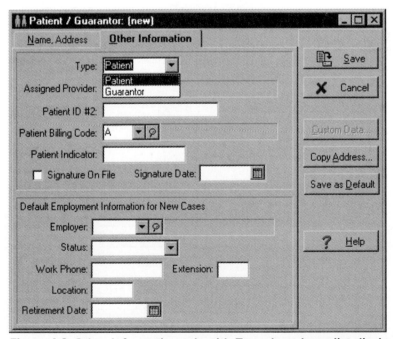

Figure 4-8 **Other Information tab with Type drop-down list displayed.**

Assigned Provider The Assigned Provider drop-down list contains codes assigned to the doctors in the practice (see Figure 4-9). The code for the specific doctor who provides care to this patient is selected.

Patient ID #2 The Patient ID #2 box is used by some medical practices as a second identification system in addition to chart numbers.

Patient Billing Code The Patient Billing Code is an optional field used to categorize patients according to the billing codes that the practice has set up in MediSoft. For example, Billing Code A might be for patients with insurance coverage, B for cash patients, and so on. Some practices use billing codes to classify patients according to a billing cycle—patients with Billing Code A are billed on the first of the month, code B on the fifteenth of the month, and so on. The Billing Code field is not used in the exercises in this book.

Patient Indicator The Patient Indicator is an optional field that practices can use to classify types of patients, such as workers' compensation patients, cash patients, diabetic patients, and so on.

Signature on File A check mark in the Signature on File check box means that the patient's signature is on file for the purpose of submitting insurance claims. This box must be completed. If it is not, insurance claims will not be accepted and processed by any insurance carrier.

Signature Date The date keyed in the Signature Date box is the date the patient signed the insurance release form.

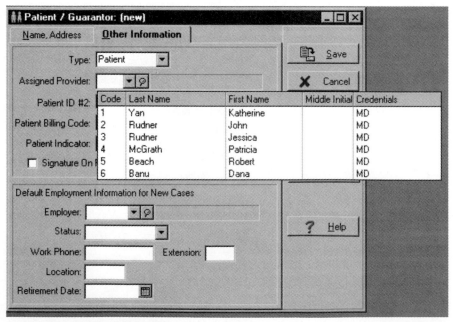

Figure 4-9 **Other Information tab with Assigned Provider drop-down list displayed.**

Employer The code for the patient's employer is selected from the drop-down list of employers that are in the database (see Figure 4-10). If the patient's employer is not in the database, this information must be entered before the code can be selected. (This process is described later in the chapter.)

Status The Status drop-down list displays the following choices for the patient's employment status: Not employed, Full time, Part time, Retired, and Unknown (see Figure 4-11).

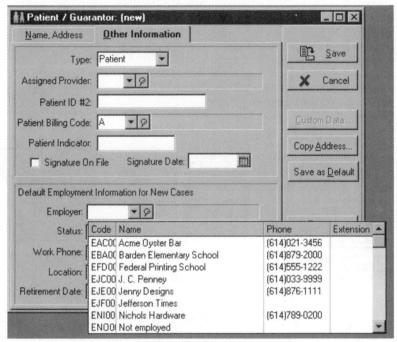

Figure 4-10 **Other Information tab with Employer drop-down list displayed.**

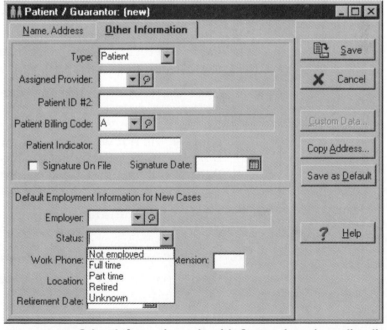

Figure 4-11 **Other Information tab with Status drop-down list displayed.**

Work Phone and Extension   Work phone numbers should be entered without parentheses or hyphens.

Location   Some companies have multiple locations. If the patient supplies information on the specific company location, it is entered in this box.

Retirement Date   The Retirement Date box is filled in only if the patient is already retired. Retirement dates should be entered in the MMDDCCYY format.

When all the fields in the Name, Address tab and the Other Information tab have been filled in, entries should be checked for accuracy. If any of the information needs to be changed, it can easily be corrected. Once the information has been checked and any necessary corrections made, data are saved by clicking the Save button.

Exercise 4-3

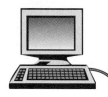

Using Source Document 1 (located in Part 4 of this book), complete the Patient/Guarantor dialog box for Hiro Tanaka, a new patient of Dr. Yan's.

1. On the Lists menu, click Patients/Guarantors and Cases, or, click the corresponding shortcut button on the toolbar.

2. Scroll down the list of patients to make sure Hiro Tanaka is not already in the patient database.

3. Click the New Patient button.

4. Create a chart number for this patient. Click the Chart Number box, and enter the chart number.

5. Click the Last Name box, and fill in the patient information. Fill in the rest of the boxes on the Name, Address tab, pressing the Tab key to move from box to box.

6. Click the Other Information tab, and fill in the appropriate boxes. Be sure to select an Assigned Provider (Dr. Yan is Tanaka's assigned provider), or subsequent exercises in this chapter will not work. The Patient ID #2 and Patient Indicator boxes should be left blank. Accept the default entry in the Patient Billing Code box. (Note: Since Tanaka's employer is not in the database, leave the employer boxes blank for now.)

7. Check your entries for accuracy, and make corrections if necessary.

8. Click the Save button to save the data on Tanaka.

9. Verify that Tanaka has been added to the list in the Patient List dialog box.

10. Close the Patient List dialog box.

ADDING AN EMPLOYER TO THE ADDRESS LIST

If the patient's employer does not appear on the Employer drop-down list in the Other Information tab, it must be entered. Addresses can be entered in one of two ways: by clicking the Addresses command on the Lists menu, or by clicking once in the Employer box on the Other Information tab and then pressing function key F8. The F8 key shortcut enables users to enter data in MediSoft in another part of the program without leaving the current dialog box. Once the F8 key is pressed, the dialog box used to enter new addresses is opened, with the Patient/Guarantor dialog box still open in the background.

When the Addresses command is clicked on the Lists menu, the Address List dialog box is displayed (see Figure 4-12). Clicking the New button at the bottom of the Address List dialog box displays the Address dialog box, just as when clicking F8 (see Figure 4-13 on page 70). Notice that clicking F8 bypassed the Address List dialog box, saving a keystroke.

The Address dialog box contains the following boxes:

Code The code for an employer should begin with the letter "E," to indicate that this is an employer. Codes can be a combination of letters and numbers, up to a maximum of five characters. If a code is not assigned, the system will assign one.

Name and Address The employer's name is entered in the Name box. This field allows up to 30 characters. The employer's street, city, state (two characters only), and zip code are entered in the boxes provided.

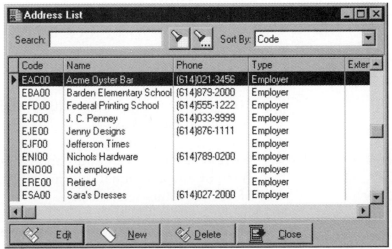

Figure 4-12 **Address List dialog box.**

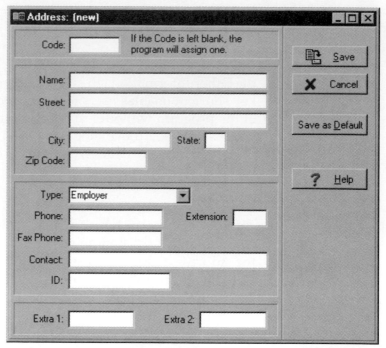

Figure 4-13 **Address dialog box.**

Type The Type drop-down list displays a list of kinds of addresses: Attorney, Employer, Facility, Laboratory, Miscellaneous, and Referral Source. For example, when the address being entered is that of an employer, "Employer" would be selected.

Phone, Extension, Fax Phone In the Phone box, the employer's phone number is entered, without parentheses or hyphens. If there is an extension, it is entered in the Extension box. The employer's fax number is entered in the Fax Phone box, also without parentheses or hyphens.

Contact The Contact box is used to enter the name of an individual at the place of employment. If there is no contact person, the box is left blank.

ID If there is an identification number for the employer, it is entered in the ID box.

Extra 1, Extra 2 The Extra 1 and Extra 2 boxes are available to keep track of any additional information that needs to be recorded and stored for future reference.

When all the information on the employer has been entered, it is saved by clicking the Save button.

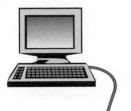

Exercise 4-4

Practice entering information about an employer.

1. Click Addresses on the Lists menu. The Address List dialog box is displayed.

2. Click the New button at the bottom of the dialog box. The Address dialog box is displayed.

3. In the Code box, key *EMCØØ* for McCray Manufacturing, Inc. ("E" for employer, followed by the first two letters of the employer's name, followed by two zeros.) Press the Tab key.

4. Key *McCray Manufacturing Inc* in the Name box. Press the Tab key.

5. In the Street box, key *1311 Kings Highway*. Press the Tab key twice.

6. Key *Stephenson* in the City box. Press the Tab key.

7. Key *OH* in the State box. Press the Tab key.

8. Key *60089* in the Zip Code box. Press the Tab key.

9. Verify that "Employer" is displayed in the Type box. If it is not, click Employer in the drop-down list and press the Tab key.

10. Key *6145550000* in the Phone box. Press the Tab key.

11. Since there is no extension or fax phone listed, leave the corresponding boxes blank.

12. Since there is no information about a contact, an ID, or any extra information, leave the corresponding boxes blank.

13. Click the Save button to store the information you have entered.

14. Click the Close button to exit the Address List dialog box.

EDITING INFORMATION ON AN ESTABLISHED PATIENT

From time to time, established patients notify the practice that they have moved, changed jobs or insurance carriers, and so on. When this happens, information needs to be updated in MediSoft's patient/guarantor database. The process of changing information on an established patient is similar to that of entering information for a new patient. The patient information is accessed through the Patient List dialog box. Then the Patients/Guarantors and Cases command is selected from the Lists menu. A search is usually performed first to locate the name or chart number of the patient whose record needs to be updated. Data can be edited either by pressing the Enter key or by clicking the Edit Patient button at the bottom of the dialog box. This displays the Patient/Guarantor dialog box, where changes can be made. Clicking the Save button stores the changes.

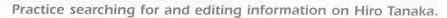

Exercise 4-5

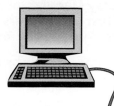

Practice searching for and editing information on Hiro Tanaka.

1. Open the Patient List dialog box.

2. Search for Hiro Tanaka by keying her chart number, *TANAKHIØ*. When the search is done, the selection arrow should be pointing to Tanaka, Hiro.

3. Click the Edit Patient button.

4. Click the Other Information tab.

5. Click the triangle button in the Employer box. Click McCray Manufacturing Inc on the drop-down list.

6. Select Full time from the Status drop-down list.

7. In the Work Phone box, key *6145551001*.

8. Click the Save button to store the information you have entered.

9. Close the Patient List dialog box.

10. Exit MediSoft.

USING TERMINOLOGY

Define the terms in the space provided.

1. chart number

_____

_____

2. guarantor

_____

_____

CHECKING YOUR UNDERSTANDING

Answer the questions below in the space provided.

3. To search for Paul Ramos, can you key either "Paul" or "Ramos"? Explain.

_____

_____

4. Create a chart number for a patient with the name of William Burroughs.

_____

5. Sam Wu has no insurance of his own but is covered by his wife's insurance policy. How would you indicate this in the Patient/Guarantor dialog box?

_____

_____

6. A patient's address is 11 West Main Street, Anytown, WI 55555. What would you enter in the City box located in the Patient/Guarantor dialog box?

_____

_____

7. How would you enter the Social Security Number 123-45-6789?

_____

APPLYING KNOWLEDGE

Answer the following question in the space provided.

8. Jane Taylor-Burke comes to the office. She thinks she saw Dr. Yan a few years ago for a flu shot, but she is not sure. You need to decide whether to enter Ms. Taylor-Burke as a new patient in the MediSoft database. What should you do?

_____

_____

_____

_____

AT THE COMPUTER

Answer the following questions at the computer:

9. How many patients in the database have the last name of Smith?

_____

10. List the name of the patient who is found when you search for the letters "JO."

_____

11. What is Li Y. Wong's chart number?

_____

12. In the Patient List dialog box, search for information on Leila Patterson. What steps did you take to find the information?

_____

_____

_____

_____

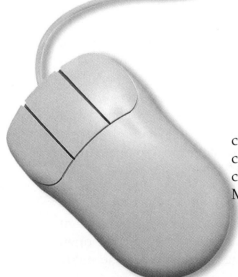

CHAPTER

5

Working with Cases

WHAT YOU NEED TO KNOW

To use this chapter, you need to know how to:
- ◆ Use the MediSoft Search feature.
- ◆ Enter new patient information.
- ◆ Locate and change information about an established patient.

OBJECTIVES

In this chapter, you will learn how to:
- ◆ Determine when to create a new case.
- ◆ Set up a new case.
- ◆ Enter information on a patient's insurance policy.
- ◆ Enter information on an accident or illness.
- ◆ Enter information on a patient's diagnosis.
- ◆ Add a new referring provider to the database.
- ◆ Add a new insurance carrier to the database.
- ◆ Edit information in an existing case.
- ◆ Close a case.
- ◆ Delete a case.

KEY TERMS

capitated plan
cases
chart
Medigap

record of treatment and progress
referring provider
sponsor

WHAT IS A CASE?

cases groupings of transactions for visits to a physician's office organized around a condition.

Cases are groupings of transactions for visits to a physician's office, organized around a condition. When a patient comes for treatment, a case is created.

Cases are set up to contain the transactions that relate to a particular condition. For example, all treatments and procedures for bronchial asthma would be stored in a case called "Bronchial asthma." Services performed and charges for those services are entered in the system and linked to the bronchial asthma case.

WHEN TO SET UP A NEW CASE

New cases should be set up each time a patient comes to see the physician for a new condition or when there is a change in the provider or insurance carrier. For example, suppose a patient has been seeing a physician regularly for treatment of bronchial asthma. All the transactions for this treatment would be contained in one case. Then suppose the patient has an accident at work and comes in for treatment of a sprained ankle. The sprained ankle is a new condition. A new case would be set up in MediSoft for the sprained-ankle treatments.

When a patient changes insurance carriers, a new case should be set up, even if the same condition is being treated under the new carrier. This makes it easier to submit insurance claims to the appropriate carrier. Transactions that took place while the previous policy was in effect must be submitted under that policy. Transactions that occur after the change in policies must be submitted to the new carrier. By opening a new case, transactions for the two insurance carriers can be kept separate. The information needed to submit claims to the previous carrier is still intact, while information for claims under the new policy is current.

A patient may require more than one case per office visit if treatment is provided for two or more unrelated conditions. For example, a patient who visits the physician complaining of migraine headaches may also ask for an influenza vaccination. Since the two conditions are unrelated, two cases would need to be created: one for the migraine headaches, and one for the vaccination. In contrast, a patient who is treated for shortness of breath and chest pain during exertion would require one case, provided the physician determines that the two complaints are related to the same diagnosis.

It is common for patients to have more than one case open at any one time. For example, in the example just mentioned, the patient would have a bronchial asthma case and a sprained-ankle case open at the same time. While the patient is being treated for the ankle injury, the bronchial asthma treatment is continuing. Some cases are for chronic conditions and remain open a long time. Other cases, such as a case for treatment of influenza NOS, may be of short duration. Cases are closed when the patient is no longer being treated for the condition, when the insurance policy in a case is no longer in effect, or when the patient leaves the practice.

CASE COMMAND BUTTONS

In MediSoft, cases are created, edited, and deleted from within the Patient List dialog box (see Figure 5-1). The Patient List dialog box is accessed by choosing Patients/Guarantors and Cases from the Lists menu. When the Case radio button in the Patient List dialog box is clicked, the following command buttons appear at the bottom of the Patient List dialog box: Edit Case, New Case, Delete Case, Copy Case, and Close (see Figure 5-2).

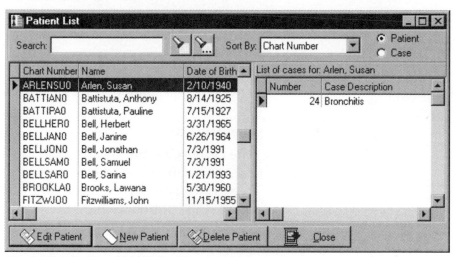

Figure 5-1 **Patient List dialog box.**

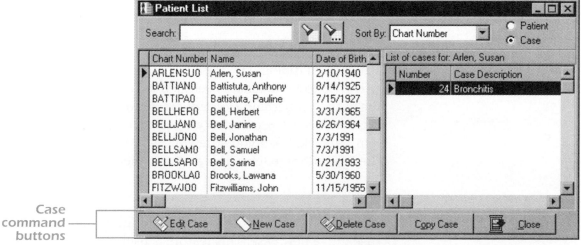

Case command buttons

Figure 5-2 **Patient List dialog box with Case radio button clicked.**

Edit Case

The Edit Case button is used to add, delete, or change information in an existing case. When the Edit Case button is clicked, the Case dialog box is displayed. Case information to be updated is contained in nine different tabs. For example, if a patient changes insurance carriers, information needs to be updated in the Policy 1, 2, or 3 tab. The only item in the Case dialog box that cannot be changed is the Case Number. All other boxes are edited by moving the cursor to the box and making the change, whether this means rekeying, selecting and deselecting a check box, or clicking a different option on a drop-down list.

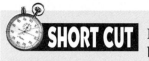 **SHORT CUT** In the Patient List dialog box, cases can also be edited by double-clicking the desired case number/description.

New Case

The New Case button creates a new case.

Delete Case

The Delete Case button deletes a case from the system if the case has no open transactions. Open transactions are charges that have not been fully paid by the insurance carrier or the policyholder. The Delete Case button should be used with caution; once deleted, information cannot be retrieved. Cases should be deleted only when it is definite that the patient's records will never be needed again. Medical offices usually have policies about when a patient's records are deleted. In most instances, it is more appropriate to close a case than to delete it from the system. Cases are closed by clicking the Case Closed box in the Personal tab of the Case folder.

When the Delete Case button is clicked, the cases are deleted in the Patient List dialog box. With the Case radio button clicked, the specific case to be deleted is selected by clicking the line that displays the case number and description. The case is then deleted by clicking the Delete Case button at the bottom of the dialog box. The system will ask, "Are you sure you want to delete this case?" Clicking the Yes button deletes the case from the system.

Copy Case

The Copy Case button copies all the information from an existing case into a new case. This feature is useful when creating a new case for a patient who already has a case in the system. Rather than reenter the information in all nine tabs, the information in the existing case is copied into a new case. Then the information that needs to be changed can be edited to reflect the data relevant to the new case. Sometimes the new case requires few changes; other times data must be changed in all the tabs of the Case folder. For this reason, it is important when copying a case to check each tab to make sure the copied information is accurate for the new case. The information that remains the same from the previous case can be left as is.

Close

The Close button closes the Patient List dialog box.

Save

After the information in all nine tabs has been checked for accuracy and edited as necessary, the case must be saved. Data recorded in the Case dialog box are stored by clicking the Save button on the right side of the Case dialog box. Clicking the Cancel button exits the Case dialog box without saving the newly entered information. The boxes that had new data entered will clear, and the screen will redisplay the Patient List dialog box.

ENTERING CASE INFORMATION

Clicking the New Case button or the Edit Case button brings up the Case dialog box. Information about a patient is entered in nine different tabs within the Case dialog box:

◆ Personal

◆ Account

◆ Diagnosis

◆ Condition

◆ Miscellaneous

◆ Policy 1

◆ Policy 2

◆ Policy 3

◆ Medicaid and Tricare

chart a folder that contains all records pertaining to a patient.

The information required to complete the nine tabs comes from documents found in a patient's chart. The **chart** is a folder that contains all records pertaining to a patient. The new patient information form supplies basic information such as name and address as well as information about insurance coverage, allergies, whether the condition is related to an accident, and the referral source. The **record of treatment and progress** contains the physician's notes about a patient's condition and diagnosis. The superbill is a list of services performed and charges for these procedures.

PERSONAL TAB

The Personal tab contains basic information about a patient and his or her employment (see Figure 5-3).

Case Number   The case number is a sequential number assigned by MediSoft. To avoid confusion, case numbers are unique; no two patients ever have the same case number.

Case Closed   A case is marked as closed by placing a check mark in the Case Closed box. At times it is appropriate to close a case. Closing a case indicates that no more data will be entered into the case. When is it appropriate to close a case? Policies vary from practice to practice, but generally cases are closed when a patient changes insurance carriers, has recovered completely from a condition (such as the flu), or is no longer a patient at the practice.

Description   Information entered in the Description box indicates a patient's complaint, or reason for seeing a physician. For example, if a patient comes to see a physician in the practice for an annual physical examination, the Description box would read "annual physical." Other examples of entries are sore throat, stomach pains, dog bite, accident at work, and so on. A patient's complaint can be found in his or her chart.

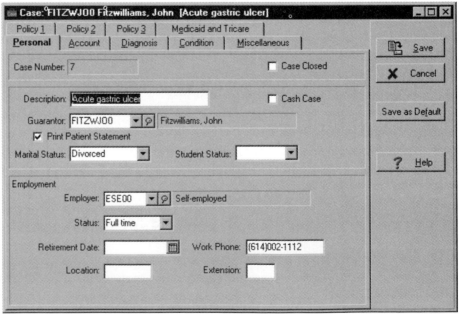

Figure 5-3 **Personal tab.**

Cash Case   If the Cash Case box is checked, the patient is paying cash and has no insurance coverage.

Guarantor   The Guarantor box lists the name of the person responsible for paying the bill. The drop-down list contains the chart numbers and names of all potential guarantors in the database.

Print Patient Statement   If this box is checked, a statement for the patient is automatically printed when statements are printed for the practice.

Marital Status   The drop-down list provides the following choices to indicate a patient's marital status: Divorced, Legally separated, Married, Single, Unknown, or Widowed.

Student Status   The Student Status drop-down list is used to indicate whether a patient is a full-time student, a part-time student, or a non-student. If a patient's status is not known, the box should be left blank.

Employer   The Employer box contains the default employer information that has been entered in the Patient/Guarantor dialog box. If it is necessary to change the employer, the default can be overridden by clicking another employer code on the drop-down list.

Status   The Status box lists a patient's employment status as it is recorded in the Patient/Guarantor dialog box. To change the selection that appears in the Status box, another selection is clicked on the drop-down list. The options are Full-time, Not employed, Part-time, Retired, and Unknown.

Retirement Date   The Retirement Date box should be filled in only when a patient is already retired. There are two ways of entering the retirement date. The date can be entered in the Retirement Date box, or it can be selected from the calendar that appears when the Pop-up Calendar button at the right of the box is clicked.

Location   If a patient has supplied a specific work location, such as "5th Avenue Branch," it is entered in the Location box.

Work Phone   The Work Phone box contains a patient's work phone number.

Extension   The Extension box lists a patient's work phone extension.

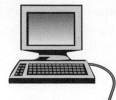

Exercise 5-1

Create a new case for patient Hiro Tanaka, and enter information in the Personal tab. The information needed to complete this exercise is found on Source Document 1.

Date: October 4, 2004

1. Start MediSoft. Change the MediSoft Program Date to the date listed above, October 4, 2004.

2. On the Lists menu, click Patients/Guarantors and Cases. The Patient List dialog box is displayed.

3. Search for Hiro Tanaka by keying TAN in the Search box. The arrow should point to the entry line for Hiro Tanaka.

4. Click the Case radio button to activate the case portion of the Patient List dialog box.

5. Click the New Case button. The dialog box labeled "Case: TANAKHI0 Tanaka, Hiro (new)" is displayed. The Personal tab is the current active tab. Notice that some information is already filled in.

6. Enter Tanaka's reason for seeing the doctor in the Description box.

7. Choose the correct entry for Tanaka's marital status from the drop-down list in the Marital Status box. The Student Status box can be left blank.

8. Notice that the information on Tanaka's employment is already filled in. The system copies the information entered in the Patient/Guarantor dialog box to the case file for you.

9. Check your entries for accuracy.

10. Click the Save button to save the case information you just entered. The Patient List dialog box redisplays. Notice that the case you just created is listed in the area of the dialog box labeled "List of cases for: Tanaka, Hiro."

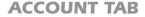

11. Do not close the Patient List dialog box.

ACCOUNT TAB   The Account tab includes information on a patient's assigned provider, referring provider, and referral source, as well as other information that may be used in some medical practices but not others (see Figure 5-4).

Assigned Provider   The Assigned Provider box is automatically filled in with the code number and name of the assigned provider listed in the Patient/Guarantor dialog box. The drop-down list provides a complete list of providers in the practice. If necessary, the Assigned Provider selection can be changed by clicking another provider on the list.

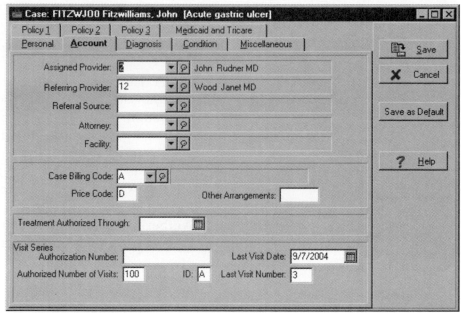

Figure 5-4 **Account tab.**

Referring Provider A **referring provider** is a physician who recommends that a patient see another specific physician. The Referring Provider box contains the name of the physician who referred the patient to the practice. The referring provider's name and code are selected from the drop-down list. If the referring provider is not listed on the drop-down list, he or she will need to be added to the Referring Provider list, which is found on the Lists menu. It is not necessary to close the Case dialog box to add a referring provider to the database. When Referring Providers is clicked on the Lists menu, the Referring Provider List dialog box opens in front of the other dialog boxes displayed on the screen. Instructions for adding a referring provider to the database are covered later in this chapter.

Referral Source If known, the source of a patient's referral is selected from the drop-down list of choices.

Attorney If a patient has an attorney, the name of the attorney should be selected from the drop-down list. If the attorney is not listed, he or she will need to be added to the system by clicking Addresses on the Lists menu and entering information about the attorney.

Facility The Facility box lists the place where a patient is receiving treatment. A facility is selected from the drop-down list. When necessary, facilities can be added to the database by clicking Addresses on the Lists menu and entering the necessary information.

Case Billing Code   The Case Billing Code box is a one- or two-character box used by some practices to classify and sort patients by insurance carrier, diagnosis, billing cycle, and so on.

Price Code   The Price Code box determines which set of fees is used when entering transactions for this case. The Price Code fees are entered and stored in the Amounts tab of the Procedure/Payment/Adjustment dialog box, accessed through the Lists menu.

Other Arrangements   If a special arrangement is made for billing, it is indicated in the Other Arrangements box.

Treatment Authorized Through   A date can be entered in this box if the insurance carrier has authorized treatment only through a certain date.

Visit Series   Information in the Visit Series section of the Account tab is used primarily by psychotherapy practices and chiropractors.

Exercise 5-2

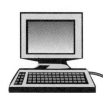

Complete the Account tab for Hiro Tanaka. The information needed to complete this exercise is found on Source Document 1.

Date: October 4, 2004

1. In the Patient List dialog box, click the line with Hiro Tanaka's name. Then click the Case radio button.

2. Click the Edit Case button to add information to Tanaka's case file. The Case dialog is displayed, with the Personal tab active.

3. Make the Account tab active. The word "Account" should now be displayed in boldfaced type, and the boxes on the Account tab should be visible.

4. Notice that the Assigned Provider box is already filled in with the name of Tanaka's assigned provider, Katherine Yan. The system copies this information from data stored in the Patient/Guarantor dialog box.

5. Click the name of Tanaka's referring provider on the Referring Provider drop-down list.

6. Notice that the entry in the Price Code box is "A." Since "A" is the list of price codes for Tanaka's insurance carrier, OhioCare HMO, you do not need to change the entry in this box.

7. Check your work for accuracy.

8. Save the changes. The Patient List dialog box is redisplayed.

9. Do not close the Patient List dialog box.

ADDING A REFERRING PROVIDER TO THE DATABASE

If a referring provider is not listed in the Referring Provider drop-down list in the Account tab, he or she will need to be added to the database. To add a referring provider, click Referring Providers on the Lists menu. The Referring Provider List dialog box is then displayed (see Figure 5-5). Clicking the New button brings up the Referring Provider dialog box, which is where information on a new referring provider is entered (see Figure 5-6). The Referring Provider dialog box contains two tabs: Address and Default Pins.

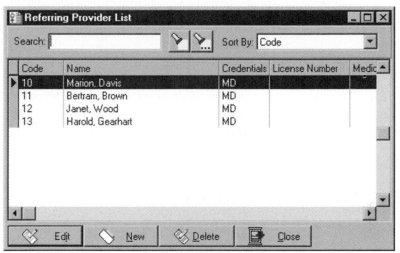

Figure 5-5 **Referring Provider List dialog box.**

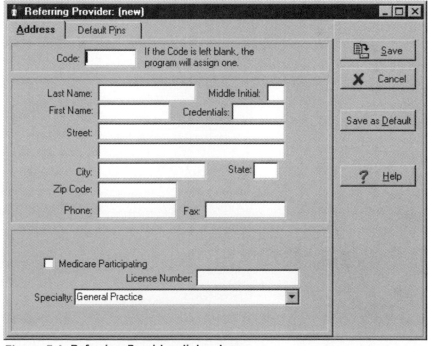

Figure 5-6 **Referring Provider dialog box.**

Address Tab

The Address tab includes a provider's name, address, license number, specialty, and Medicare participation status (see Figure 5-7).

Code The Code box contains a unique identification code assigned to a referring provider. It can be up to five characters. If a code is not entered in the Code box, the system will assign one.

Name, Address, and Phone Numbers The Last Name, Middle Initial, First Name, Street, City, State, Zip Code, Phone, and Fax boxes list basic information about a referring provider.

Credentials The Credentials box lists a referring provider's professional credentials, such as MD, DO, PhD, RN, and so on. This box can be up to three characters long.

Medicare Participating If a referring provider is a participating Medicare provider, the Medicare Participating box is checked.

License Number A referring provider's license number is listed in the License Number box.

Specialty A referring provider's specialty is selected from the corresponding drop-down list. If the specialty is not one of the choices on the list, click the category "All other."

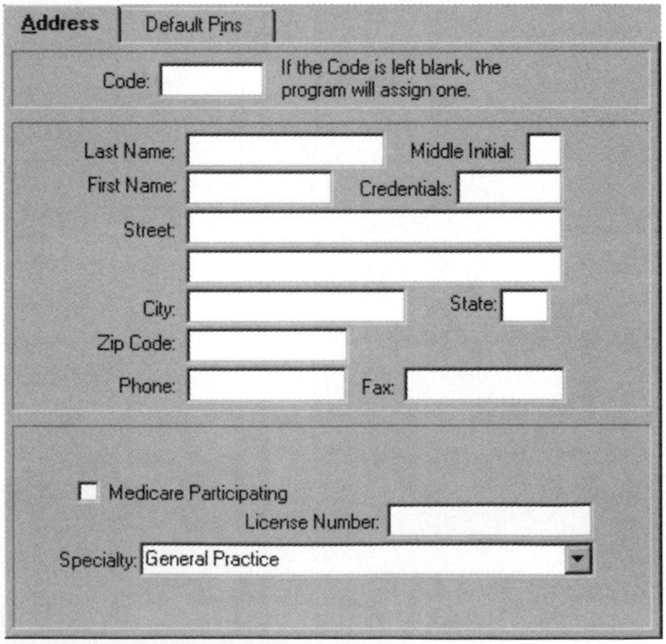

Figure 5-7 **Address tab.**

Default Pins Tab

The Default Pins tab contains identification numbers assigned to a referring provider (see Figure 5-8).

SSN/Federal Tax ID   The SSN/Federal Tax ID box contains a provider's Social Security number or Federal Tax Identification number. If the Federal Tax Identification number is entered, the box labeled "Federal Tax ID Indicator" should also be checked.

PINs   In the boxes listed, a referring provider's PINs (provider identification numbers) are entered for each insurance type: Medicare, Medicaid, Tricare, Blue Cross/Shield, Commercial, PPO, and HMO.

UPIN   The provider's Unique Physician Identifier Number (UPIN) is entered in the UPIN box.

Extra 1, Extra 2   These boxes can be used to enter any additional information about the referring provider.

EMC ID   The EMC ID box contains the identification number assigned to a physician by the EMC clearinghouse.

When all the information about the referring provider has been entered and checked for accuracy, it is saved by clicking the Save button in the Referring Provider dialog box.

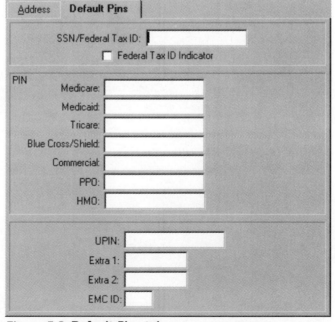

Figure 5-8 **Default Pins tab.**

DIAGNOSIS TAB The Diagnosis tab contains a patient's diagnosis, information about allergies, and electronic media claim (EMC) notes (see Figure 5-9).

Diagnosis 1 through Diagnosis 4   A patient's diagnosis is selected from the drop-down list of diagnoses. If a patient has more than one diagnosis, the primary diagnosis is entered as Diagnosis 1. Up to four diagnoses can be entered for each case. If there are more than four diagnoses, a new case must be opened.

Allergies and Notes   If a patient has allergies or any other special condition that needs to be recorded, they are entered in the Allergies and Notes box.

EMC Notes   If a patient's claims require special handling when submitted electronically, notes about the procedure, such as an explanation about the charges for supplies, are listed in this box.

Exercise 5-3

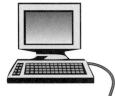

Complete the Diagnosis tab for Hiro Tanaka. The information needed to complete this exercise is found on Source Documents 1 and 2.

Date: October 4, 2004

1. **Edit the case for Hiro Tanaka.**

2. **Make the Diagnosis tab active.**

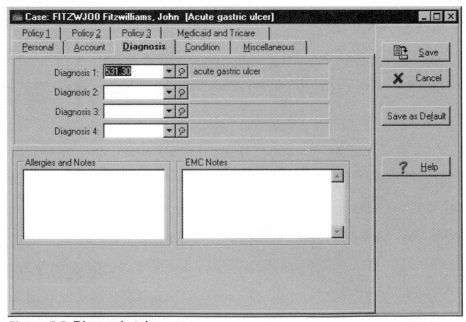

Figure 5-9 **Diagnosis tab.**

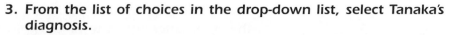

3. **From the list of choices in the drop-down list, select Tanaka's diagnosis.**

4. **In the Allergies and Notes box, enter information on Tanaka's allergies.**

5. **Check your work for accuracy.**

6. **Save the changes. The Patient List dialog box is redisplayed.**

7. **Do not close the Patient List dialog box.**

CONDITION TAB   The Condition tab stores data about a patient's illness, accident, disability, and hospitalization (see Figure 5-10). This information is used by insurance carriers to process claims.

Injury/Illness/LMP Date   The date of a patient's injury, illness, or last menstrual period (LMP) is entered in the Injury/Illness/LMP Date box. (For an illness, the date when the symptoms first appeared is entered.)

Illness Indicator   The Illness Indicator box specifies whether a patient's condition is an illness or a last menstrual period, in the case of a pregnancy.

First Consultation Date   The date of a patient's first visit for a particular condition is entered in the First Consultation Date box. The actual date can be entered, or the pop-up calendar can be activated and dates selected from the calendar.

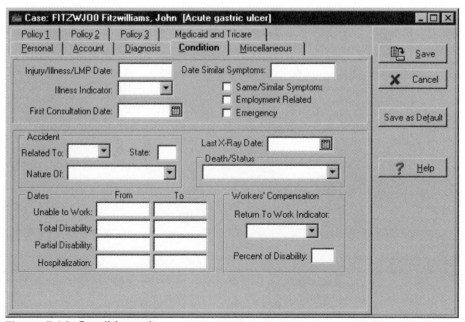

Figure 5-10 **Condition tab.**

Date Similar Symptoms   If a patient has had similar symptoms in the past, enter the date of those symptoms in the Date Similar Symptoms box.

Same/Similar Symptoms   A check mark in the Same/Similar Symptoms box indicates that a patient has had the same or similar symptoms in the past.

Employment Related   If the Employment Related box is checked, it means that the illness or accident is in some way related to a patient's employment.

Emergency   If a patient sees the provider on an emergency visit, a check mark is entered in the Emergency box.

Accident—Related To   The Accident—Related To box indicates whether a patient's condition is related to an accident. The drop-down list offers three choices: Auto, if it is related to an automobile accident; No, if it is not accident-related; and Yes, if it is accident-related but not an auto accident. If a patient's condition is accident-related, the State and Nature Of boxes should also be completed.

Accident—State   The abbreviation for the state in which the accident occurred is entered in this box.

Accident—Nature Of   This box provides additional information about the type of accident. The following choices can be selected from the drop-down list: Injured at home, Injured at school, Injured during recreation, Motorcycle injury, Work injury/Non-collision, and Work injury/Self employed.

Dates—Unable to Work   If a patient is unable to work, the dates of the absence from work are listed in these boxes.

Dates—Total Disability   If a patient is totally disabled, the dates of the total disability are entered in these boxes.

Dates—Partial Disability   If a patient is partially disabled, the dates of the partial disability are listed in these boxes.

Dates—Hospitalization   If a patient is hospitalized, the dates of the hospitalization are entered in these boxes.

Last X-Ray Date   The Last X-Ray Date box is used by chiropractic offices to list the date of a patient's last X ray.

Death/Status   The Death/Status box indicates a patient's condition according to the Karnofsky Performance Status Scale. There are 11 options: Able to carry on normal activity, Cares for self, Dead, Disabled, Moribund (a terminal condition near death), Normal, Normal activity with effort, Requires considerable assistance, Requires occasional assistance, Severely disabled, and Very sick. If this information is not provided by the physician, the box should be left blank.

Workers' Compensation—Return to Work Indicator If a patient has been out of work on Workers' Compensation, the patient's return to work status is selected from the drop-down list of choices: Conditional, Limited, or Normal. If the status is Conditional or Limited, the Percent of Disability box should also be completed.

Workers' Compensation—Percent of Disability This box indicates a patient's percent of disability upon returning to work

Exercise 5-4

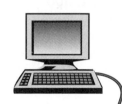

Complete the Condition tab for Hiro Tanaka. The information needed to complete this exercise is found on Source Documents 1 and 3.

Date: October 4, 2004

1. Edit the case for Hiro Tanaka.

2. Make the Condition tab active.

3. Enter the date of the injury in the Injury/Illness/LMP Date box.

4. Leave the Illness Indicator box blank.

5. In the First Consultation Date box, enter the date Tanaka first saw Dr. Yan for this condition.

6. Since this visit resulted from a non-work-related accident, leave the Date Similar Symptoms box, the Same/Similar Symptoms box, and the Employment Related box blank.

7. Since this was an emergency visit, place a check mark in the Emergency box by clicking it.

8. Choose Auto in the Accident—Related To box.

9. In the Accident—State box, enter the two-letter abbreviation for the state in which the accident occurred.

10. Tanaka was injured while driving home from a softball game. Complete the Accident—Nature Of box regarding the type of accident with Injured during Recreation.

11. Enter the dates Tanaka was unable to work in the Dates— Unable to Work boxes.

12. Enter the dates Tanaka was totally disabled in the Dates—Total Disability boxes.

13. Enter the dates Tanaka was partially disabled in the Dates—Partial Disability boxes.

14. Enter the dates Tanaka was hospitalized in the Dates—Hospitalization boxes.

15. Leave the Last X-Ray Date box blank.

16. Since Tanaka was not injured at work, the Workers' Compensation boxes should be left blank.

17. Check your work for accuracy.

18. Save the changes.

19. Do not close the Patient List dialog box.

MISCELLANEOUS TAB

The Miscellaneous tab records a variety of miscellaneous information about the patient and his or her treatment (see Figure 5-11).

Outside Lab Work If the Outside Lab Work box is checked, the lab work was performed by a lab other than the physician's office. If the lab bills the provider rather than the patient, then the provider bills the patient for the lab work even though it was performed by an outside lab.

Lab Charges The charges for lab work, whether performed inside or outside the practice, are entered in the Lab Charges box.

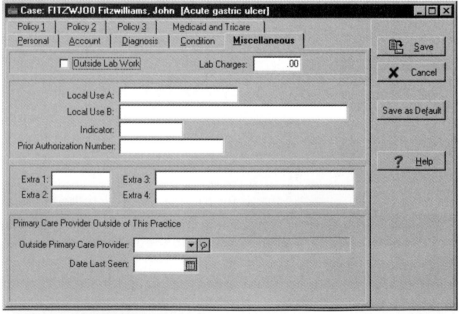

Figure 5-11 **Miscellaneous tab.**

Local Use A and B   These boxes may be used by some medical practices to record information specific to the local office.

Indicator   If an indicator code is used to categorize patients or services, it is entered in the Indicator box. For example, patients might be categorized according to their primary diagnosis. Services might be divided into such categories as lab work, consultations, hospital visits, and so on.

Prior Authorization Number   Before some services are performed, prior authorization must be obtained from the appropriate insurance carrier. If an insurance carrier has issued an authorization number for treatment that has not yet occurred, the number is entered in the Prior Authorization Number box.

Extra 1, 2, 3, and 4   The Extra 1, 2, 3, and 4 boxes are used for different purposes depending on the medical practice.

Primary Care Provider Outside of This Practice   If a patient is covered by a managed care plan and the patient's primary care provider is outside the medical practice, the name of the provider is selected from the drop-down list in this box.

Date Last Seen   The Date Last Seen box lists the date a patient was last seen by the outside primary care provider.

POLICY 1 TAB   The Policy 1 tab is where information about a patient's primary insurance carrier and coverage is recorded (see Figure 5-12).

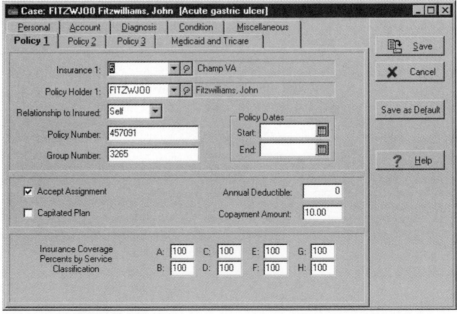

Figure 5-12 **Policy 1 tab.**

Insurance 1   The Insurance 1 box lists the code number and name of the insurance carrier. The drop-down list provides a list of carriers already in the system. If the carrier is not listed, it must be added to the database. It is not necessary to close the Case dialog box to add an insurance carrier to the database. When Insurance Carriers is clicked on the Lists menu, the Insurance Carrier List dialog box is displayed in front of the other dialog boxes on the screen. Instructions for adding an insurance carrier to the database are covered later in this chapter.

Policy Holder 1   The Policy Holder box lists the person who is the insured for a particular policy. For example, if the patient is a child covered under his or her parent's insurance plan, the parent's chart number would be entered in this box. The insured's chart number is selected from the choices on the drop-down list. (If the insured is not a patient of the practice, he or she must be entered as a guarantor in MediSoft, and a chart number must be established.)

Relationship to Insured   This box describes a patient's relationship to the individual listed in the Insured 1 box. The drop-down list offers the following choices: Child, Other, Self, and Spouse.

Policy Number   A patient's policy number is entered in the Policy Number box.

Group Number   The group number for a patient's policy is entered in the Group Number box.

Policy Dates—Start/End   The date a patient's insurance policy went into effect is entered in the Policy Dates—Start box. If the date is not known, the date the patient first came to the practice for treatment can be entered. If the policy has ended, such as when the carrier changes or when the coverage expires, the date on which coverage terminated is entered in the Policy Dates—End box.

Accept Assignment   For physicians who are participating in an insurance plan, a check mark in the Accept Assignment box indicates that the provider accepts payment directly from the insurance carrier.

capitated plan an insurance plan in which payments are made to primary care providers for patients, regardless of whether or not they visit the provider during the stated time period.

Capitated Plan   In a **capitated plan**, payments are made to physicians from managed care companies for patients who select the physician as their primary care provider, regardless of whether they visit the physician or not. A check mark in this box indicates that this insurance plan is capitated.

Annual Deductible   The dollar amount of the insured's insurance plan deductible is entered in this box.

Copayment Amount   The dollar amount of a patient's copayment per visit is entered in the Copayment Amount box.

Insurance Coverage Percents by Service Classification   The percentage of fees that an insurance carrier covers is entered in the Insurance Coverage Percents by Service Classification box. Some insurance plans pay different percentages of charges based on the type of service provided. For example, a plan may pay 80 percent of necessary medical procedures and 50 percent of outpatient mental health charges. A practice can assign a different category of service to each of the letters A through H. For example, "A" could represent necessary medical procedures performed in the office, "B" could represent preventive procedures, "C" laboratory tests, "D" outpatient mental health services, and so on. With some managed care plans, 100 percent is entered in boxes A through H, because the patient is required to pay a copayment only, not a percentage of the charges.

ADDING AN INSURANCE CARRIER TO THE DATABASE

If an insurance carrier is not listed in the Insurance drop-down list in the Policy 1, 2, or 3 tabs, it needs to be added to the database. To add an insurance carrier, click Insurance Carriers on the Lists menu. The Insurance Carrier List dialog box lists all the carriers already in the system (see Figure 5-13). Clicking the New button brings up the Insurance Carrier (new) dialog box, where information on a carrier is entered (see Figure 5-14 on page 96). The Insurance Carrier (new) dialog box contains five tabs: Address; Options; EMC, Codes; Allowed; and PINs.

Address Tab

The Address tab contains basic information about an insurance carrier (again, see Figure 5-14 on page 96).

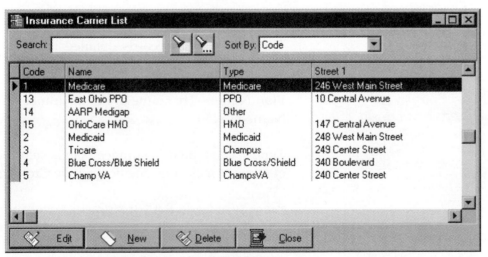

Figure 5-13 **Insurance Carrier List dialog box.**

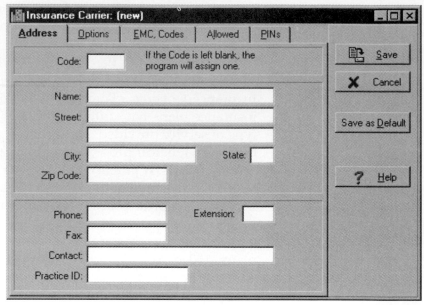

Figure 5-14 **Insurance Carrier (new) dialog box.**

Code The code is a unique identification number assigned to an insurance carrier. It can be up to five characters long. If a code is not entered in the Code box, the system will assign one.

Name, Address, and Phone Numbers The Name, Street, City, State, Zip Code, Phone, Extension, and Fax boxes list basic information about a carrier.

Contact If there is a specific person at the insurance carrier who is assigned to handle the practice's claims, that person's name is entered in the Contact box.

Practice ID The Practice ID box lists the identification number assigned to the practice by the insurance carrier.

Options Tab

The Options tab records detailed information about an insurance carrier (see Figure 5-15).

Plan Name The name of the insurance plan is entered in the Plan Name box.

Type The type of insurance plan is selected from a drop-down list of choices, including Medicare, Blue Cross/Shield, HMO, and so on.

Procedure Code Set If a practice uses more than one set of procedure codes, enter the code number for the set used by the particular insurance carrier.

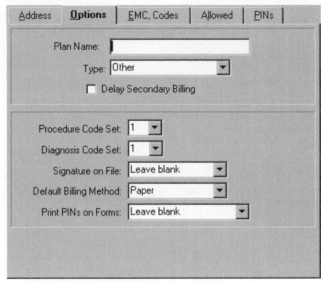

Figure 5-15 **Options tab.**

Diagnosis Code Set   If a practice uses more than one set of diagnosis codes, enter the code number for the set used by the particular insurance carrier.

Signature on File   The Signature on File box controls whether a patient's signature is printed on an insurance claim form to indicate that he or she has authorized payment to be sent directly to the provider. The choices on the drop-down list are Leave blank, Signature on file, and Print name.

Default Billing Method   The Default Billing Method box indicates whether claims are to be submitted electronically or on paper. For the purposes of this book, the default method for submitting claims is electronic.

Print PINs on Forms   The Print PINs on Forms box indicates whether the provider name and PINs are to be printed on claim forms.

EMC, Codes Tab

The third tab in the Insurance Carrier (new) dialog box is the EMC, Codes tab. This tab contains information on electronic media claims (see Figure 5-16 on page 98).

EMC Receiver   The EMC Receiver box contains the name of the receiver of electronic media claims for a particular insurance carrier.

EMC Payor Number   The payor identification number assigned by the clearinghouse is entered in the EMC Payor Number box.

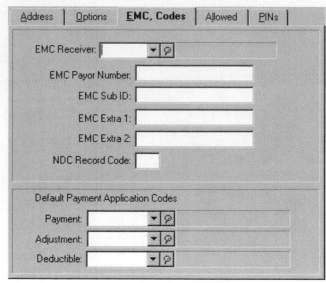

Figure 5-16 **EMC, Codes tab.**

EMC Sub ID   The EMC Sub ID box contains the sub ID number assigned by the clearinghouse.

EMC Extra 1 and 2   The EMC Extra 1 and EMC Extra 2 boxes can be used to enter additional information about the EMC setup.

NDC Record Code   The record code assigned by the clearinghouse is entered in the NDC (National Data Corporation) Record Code box.

When all the information on an insurance carrier has been entered and checked for accuracy, data is saved by clicking the Save button.

Allowed Tab

The next tab in the Insurance Carrier (new) dialog box is the Allowed tab (see Figure 5-17). This tab lists all procedure codes in the MediSoft database and this insurance carrier's allowed amount for each procedure. The program automatically completes the boxes in the Allowed column when insurance payments are applied to procedures (this is covered in Chapter 7).

PINs Tab

The last tab in the Insurance Carrier (new) dialog box is the PINs tab (see Figure 5-18). This tab lists the insurance carrier's assigned PIN and Group ID for each provider in the practice.

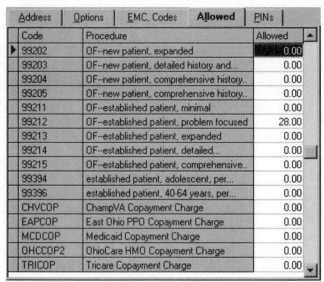

Figure 5-17 **Allowed tab.**

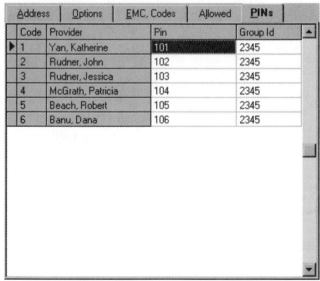

Figure 5-18 **PINs tab.**

Exercise 5-5

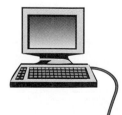

Complete the Policy 1 tab for Hiro Tanaka. The information needed to complete this exercise is found on Source Document 1.

Date: October 4, 2004

1. Edit the case for Hiro Tanaka.

2. Make the Policy 1 tab active.

3. Select Tanaka's primary insurance carrier from the drop-down list in the Insurance 1 box.

4. Select the chart number and name of the person who should be entered in the Policy Holder 1 box from the list of choices in the drop-down list.

5. Notice that the Relationship to Insured box already has "Self" entered. If this is correct, do not make any changes. If it is incorrect, make another selection from the drop-down list.

6. Enter Tanaka's insurance policy number in the Policy Number box.

7. Enter Tanaka's group number in the Group Number box.

8. In the Policy Dates—Start box, key *10012004* as the start date of the policy.

9. Dr. Yan accepts assignment for this carrier, so click the Accept Assignment box.

10. The insurance plan is capitated, so check the Capitated Plan box.

11. Key *15* in the Copayment box if it does not already appear in the box.

12. Key *100* in each of the Insurance Coverage Percents by Service Classification boxes.

13. Check your work for accuracy.

14. Save the changes.

15. Do not close the Patient List dialog box.

POLICY 2 TAB   The boxes in the Policy 2 tab are the same as those in the Policy 1 tab, with a few exceptions. The Copayment Amount and Capitated Plan boxes are only in the Policy 1 tab. Only the Policy 2 tab has a Crossover Claim box (see Figure 5-19).

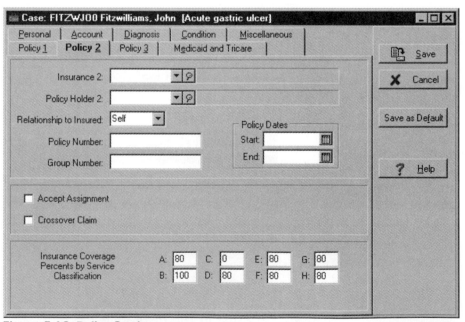

Figure 5-19 **Policy 2 tab.**

Crossover Claim   The Crossover Claim box is used to indicate an insurance plan such as a Medigap policy. **Medigap** is a supplementary insurance plan offered by a private insurance company that is designed to supplement Medicare. Because Medicare is the primary carrier, it pays first on a claim and then submits the claim to the Medigap carrier. If the Crossover Claim box is checked, it indicates that Policy 2 is a Medigap plan.

POLICY 3 TAB

The Policy 3 tab does not contain the Copayment Amount, Capitated Plan, and Crossover Claim boxes. Otherwise, the boxes are the same as those in the Policy 1 and Policy 2 tabs (see Figure 5-20).

MEDICAID AND TRICARE TAB

For patients covered by Medicaid or TRICARE, the Medicaid and Tricare tab is used to enter additional information about the government programs (see Figure 5-21 on page 102).

Medicaid

EPSDT   EPSDT stands for "Early and Periodic Screening, Diagnosis, and Treatment." This is a Medicaid program for patients under the age of 21 who need screening and diagnostic services to determine physical or mental problems as well as treatment for conditions discovered. It also includes well-baby checkup examinations. A check mark in the EPSDT box indicates that a patient's visit is part of the EPSDT program.

Family Planning   A check mark in the Family Planning box specifies that a patient's condition is related to family planning.

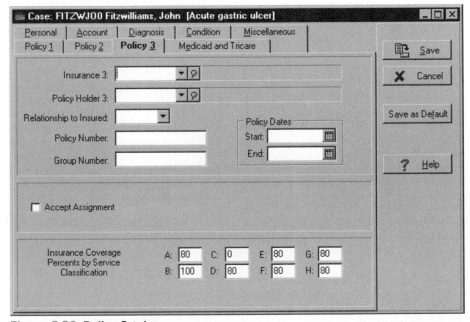

Figure 5-20 **Policy 3 tab.**

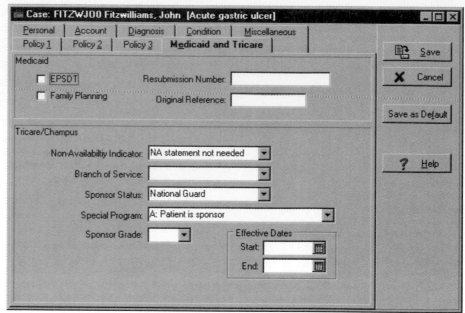

Figure 5-21 **Medicaid and TRICARE tab.**

Resubmission Number   For claims being resubmitted to Medicaid, the resubmission number is entered in this box.

Original Reference   For claims being resubmitted to Medicaid, the original reference number is recorded in the Original Reference box.

TRICARE

TRICARE is the government insurance program that serves spouses and children of active-duty service members, military retirees and their families, some former spouses, and survivors of deceased military members (Army, Navy, Air Force, Marine Corps, Coast Guard, Public Health Service, and the National Oceanic and Atmospheric Administration).

Non-Availability Indicator   The Non-Availability Indicator box specifies whether a nonavailability statement is required. The choices on the drop-down list are NA statement not needed, NA statement obtained, and Other carrier paid at least 75%.

Branch of Service   The Branch of Service box indicates the particular branch of service: Air Force, Army, CHAMPVA, Coast Guard, Marines, Navy, NOAA, and Public Health Service.

sponsor an active-duty service member.

Sponsor Status   The **sponsor** is the active-duty service member. The sponsor's family members are covered by the TRICARE insurance plan. The drop-down list in the Sponsor Status box provides choices to indicate the sponsor's status in the service, such as Active, Medal of Honor, Reserves, and so on.

Effective Dates The start date of the TRICARE policy is entered in the Effective Dates—Start box. If there is an end date, it is entered in the Effective Dates—End box. Specific dates can be entered, or a selection can be made from the pop-up calendar.

Special Program The Special Program drop-down list contains codes for special TRICARE programs.

Sponsor Grade The two-character sponsor grade is entered in the Sponsor Grade box.

EDITING CASE INFORMATION ON AN ESTABLISHED PATIENT

Information in an existing case is modified by selecting the case to be edited and clicking the Edit Case button at the bottom of the Patient List dialog box. (The Case radio button must be clicked for the Edit Case button to be displayed.)

Exercise 5-6

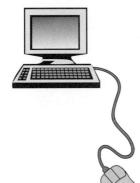

John Fitzwilliams, an established patient, has just remarried. Edit the information in his Case dialog box to reflect this change.

Date: October 4, 2004

1. In the Personal tab, change the entry in the Marital Status box from Divorced to Married.

2. Check your work for accuracy.

3. Save the changes.

4. Close the Patient List dialog box.

5. Exit MediSoft.

CHAPTER REVIEW

USING TERMINOLOGY

Match the terms on the left with the definitions on the right.

_____ 1. capitated plan

_____ 2. cases

_____ 3. chart

_____ 4. Medigap

_____ 5. record of treatment and progress

_____ 6. referring provider

_____ 7. sponsor

a. A folder that contains a patient's medical records.

b. Physician's notes about a patient's condition and diagnosis.

c. A physician who recommends that a patient make an appointment with a particular doctor.

d. A private insurance plan that supplements Medicare coverage.

e. An insurance plan in which payments are made to primary care providers for patients whether they have an office visit or not.

f. Groupings of transactions organized around a patient's condition.

g. The active-duty service member on the TRICARE government insurance program.

CHECKING YOUR UNDERSTANDING

Answer the questions below in the space provided.

8. Sarina Bell has no insurance of her own but is covered by her father's insurance policy. How would this be indicated in the Policy 1 tab for Sarina Bell?

_____

_____

9. Where in the Case dialog box can you find information about a patient's allergies?

_____

_____

10. Is it necessary to set up a new case when a patient changes insurance carriers? Why?

_____

_____

11. In the Case dialog box, where would you enter information about a work-related accident?

_____

_____

12. Where is information needed to complete the Diagnosis tab usually found?

_____

_____

13. A patient has been seeing the doctor regularly for treatment of diabetes. She was hospitalized yesterday, and the doctor saw her in the hospital for treatment. Do you need to set up a new case for the hospitalization?

_____

_____

APPLYING KNOWLEDGE

Answer the questions below in the space provided.

14. While you are entering case information for a new patient, you realize that the patient's referring provider is not one of the choices in the Referring Provider box in the Account tab. What should you do?

_____

_____

15. One of the established patients has changed insurance carriers from Blue Cross/ Blue Shield to OhioCare HMO. What specific boxes need to be changed in the Case dialog box?

_____

_____

AT THE COMPUTER

Answer the following questions at the computer:

16. Using the information contained in the Case dialog box, list Randall Klein's primary and secondary insurance carriers.

_____

_____

17. Who is the guarantor for Janine Bell's account?

_____

6 Entering Charge Transactions

WHAT YOU NEED TO KNOW

To use this chapter, you need to know how to:
◆ Start MediSoft, use menus, and enter and edit text.
◆ Edit information in an existing case.
◆ Work with chart and case numbers.

OBJECTIVES

In this chapter, you will learn how to:
◆ Record information about patients' visits, including procedure codes and charges.
◆ Edit charge transactions.
◆ Use MediSoft's Search features to find specific transaction data.

KEY TERMS

adjustments   MultiLink codes
charges   payments
modifiers

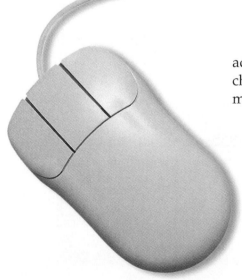

TRANSACTION ENTRY OVERVIEW

charges the amounts a provider bills for services performed.

payments monies received from patients and insurance carriers.

adjustments changes to patients' accounts.

Three types of transactions are recorded in MediSoft: charges, payments, and adjustments. **Charges** are the amounts a provider bills for the services performed. **Payments** are monies received from patients and insurance carriers. **Adjustments** are changes to patients' accounts. Examples of adjustments include returned check fees, insurance write-offs, Medicare adjustments, and changes in treatment. This chapter covers charge transactions. Chapter 7 covers payment and adjustment transactions.

The primary document needed to enter charge transactions in Medi-Soft is a patient's superbill (also called a charge ticket or encounter form). Typically, the physician circles or checks the appropriate procedure and diagnosis codes on the superbill during or just after the patient visit. Charges and payments listed on a superbill are later entered in the Transaction Entry dialog box in MediSoft by an insurance billing specialist. After the information is entered, it is checked for accuracy. If all the information is correct, the transaction data are saved and a walkout receipt is printed for the patient. If it is incorrect, the data are edited and then saved.

THE TRANSACTION ENTRY DIALOG BOX

Transactions are entered in the Transaction Entry dialog box, which is accessed by clicking Enter Transactions on the Activities menu (see Figure 6-1). The Transaction Entry dialog box lists existing transac-

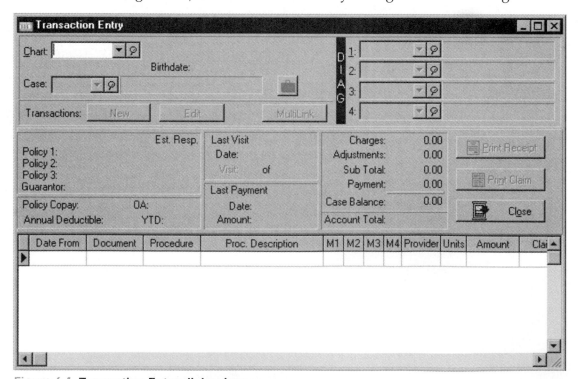

Figure 6-1 **Transaction Entry dialog box.**

tions and provides options for editing existing transactions and creating new transactions. The following section provides an overview of the different areas of the Transaction Entry dialog box.

All transactions entered in MediSoft begin with two critical pieces of information: a patient's chart number and the case number, which is related to the procedures performed. The chart number and case number must be selected in the Transaction Entry dialog box before a transaction can be entered. Boxes for entering these numbers are found at the top left of the dialog box.

Chart To begin entering a new transaction, a patient's chart number is selected on the drop-down list in the Chart box. Many practices have long lists of chart numbers in MediSoft. The fastest way to enter a chart number is to key the first few letters of the patient's last name, which then displays that location in the drop-down list of chart numbers.

Case After the chart number has been selected, the Case box displays a case number and description for a particular patient (see Figure 6-2). If a patient has more than one open case, the drop-down list displays the full list of cases. Only one case can be opened at a time. The transactions listed at the bottom of the dialog box pertain to the particular case selected in the Case box. Transactions for other cases can be displayed by changing the selection in the Case box.

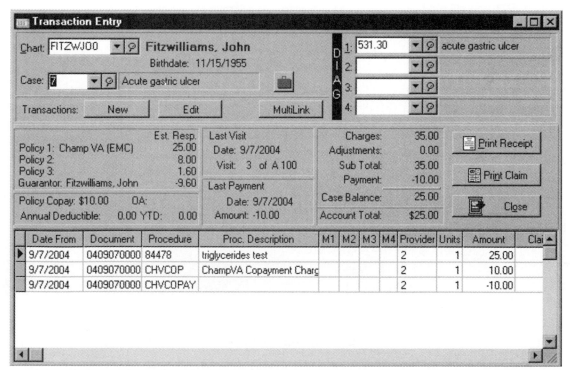

Figure 6-2 **Transaction Entry dialog box with case data displayed.**

After the chart and case numbers have been entered, a new transaction can be created or an existing transaction can be edited. Transactions already in the system for a patient whose chart number is active are listed at the bottom of the dialog box. The scroll bar at the bottom of the dialog box may be used to display a full summary of the transaction (see Figure 6-3).

The process of creating a new transaction in MediSoft begins with clicking the New button. When the New button is clicked, three transaction entry tabs appear: Charge, Payment, and Adjustment. (Payments and adjustments are described in Chapter 7.)

ENTERING CHARGES

Charges for procedures are entered in the Charge tab (see Figure 6-4). This tab contains the following boxes:

Dates   In the Dates boxes, the system automatically defaults to the current date, that is, the MediSoft Program Date. If this is not the date on which the procedures were performed, the data in the Dates boxes need to be changed to reflect the actual date of the procedures. Data in these boxes can be changed by keying over the information that is already there. New dates can also be selected by clicking the pop-up calendar buttons beside the Dates boxes.

To change the default date for these boxes, either of these methods is used:

◆   The Set Program Date command on the File menu is clicked, or

◆   The date button in the bottom right corner of the screen is clicked. (This must be done before the New button is clicked in the Transaction Entry dialog box.)

Document   The system displays a document number automatically; it is the current date (listed in YYMMDD format instead of the usual MMDDYY format) followed by four zeros. Some medical offices use document numbers, others do not. One common use of the Document field is to record the superbill number that lists the procedures performed. Up to 10 characters can be entered. For the

Bill 1	Bill 2	Bill 3	Statement	Visit#	Visit ID	Description	Place of Service	Case Number	Chart Number
				3	A		11	7	FITZWJ00
				3	A		11	7	FITZWJ00
				0				/	ᴬᴺ. 0

Figure 6-3 **Information displayed when scrolling to the right.**

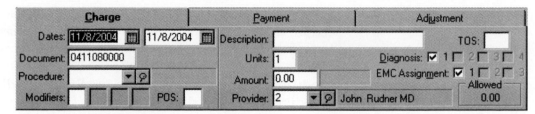

Figure 6-4 **Charge tab.**

purposes of this book, use the default document numbers assigned by the system.

Procedure The procedure code for a service performed is selected from the drop-down list of CPT codes already entered in the system. Only one procedure code can be selected for each transaction. If multiple procedures were performed for a patient, each one must be entered as a separate transaction, or a MultiLink code, which is discussed in the next paragraph, must be used. After the code is selected from the drop-down list and the Tab key or Enter key is pressed, the charge for a procedure is displayed in the Amount box. If a CPT code is not listed, it will need to be added to the database by pressing the F8 key or by clicking Procedure/Payment/Adjustment Codes on the Lists menu. This may be done without exiting the Transaction Entry dialog box.

MULTILINK CODES

MultiLink codes *groups of procedure code entries that relate to a single activity.*

MediSoft provides a feature that saves time when entering multiple CPT codes that are related. **MultiLink codes** are groups of procedure code entries that relate to a single activity. Using MultiLink codes saves time by eliminating the need to enter related multiple procedure codes one at a time. For example, suppose a MultiLink code is created for the procedures related to diagnosing a strep throat. The MultiLink code STREPM is created. STREPM includes three procedures: 99211 Minimal Visit, 87072 Strep Culture, and 85022 CBC w/Diff.

When the MultiLink code STREPM is selected, all three procedure codes are entered automatically by the system, eliminating the need to make three different entries. The MultiLink feature saves time by reducing the number of procedure code entries, and it also reduces omission errors. When procedure codes are entered as a MultiLink, it is impossible to forget to enter a procedure, since all of the codes that are in the MultiLink group are entered automatically.

MultiLink

Figure 6-5 **MultiLink button.**

Clicking the MultiLink button (see Figure 6-5) in the Transaction Entry dialog box displays the MultiLink dialog box. After a MultiLink code is selected from the MultiLink drop-down list, the Create

Transactions button is clicked. The codes and charges for each procedure are automatically added to the list of transactions at the bottom of the Transaction Entry dialog box.

Modifiers   Some CPT codes use modifiers. **Modifiers** are one- or two-digit codes that allow a more specific description to be entered for the services the physician performed. For example, a modifier needs to be used when the circumstances require services beyond those normally associated with a particular procedure code. A common modifier is -90, which indicates that the procedure is performed by an outside laboratory. If a modifier is indicated on a superbill, it is entered in the Modifiers box. MediSoft permits up to four modifiers for each procedure code.

POS   The POS, or Place of Service box, indicates where services were performed. The standard numerical codes used are:

11   Provider's office

21   Inpatient hospital

22   Outpatient hospital

23   Hospital emergency room

When MediSoft is set up for use in a practice, an option is provided to set a default POS code. In addition, POS codes can be assigned to specific procedure codes when they are set up in the Procedure/Payment/Adjustment List. For purposes of this book, the default code has been set to 11 for Provider's office.

Description   The Description box is normally left blank in the Charge tab. It can be used to enter a brief note for internal use. The field does not print on any claims or reports.

Units   The Units box indicates the quantity of the procedure. Normally, the number of units is one. In some cases, however, it may be more than one. For example, if a patient was seen by a physician for three days of hospital visits and the charge linked to the CPT code is for one day, "3" would be entered in the Units box.

Amount   The Amount box lists the charge amount for a procedure. The amount is entered automatically by the system based on the CPT code and insurance carrier. Each CPT code stored in the system has a charge amount associated with it for each insurance carrier. The charge amount can be edited if necessary. To the right of the Amount box is the Extended Amount area. This area displays the total charges for the procedure(s) performed. The amount is calculated by the system; the number in the Units box is multiplied by the number in the Amount box. For example, suppose a patient had three X rays done at a charge of $45.00 per X ray. The Units box would read "3," and the Amount box would read "$45.00." The Extended Amount box would read "$135.00," which is 3 x $45.00.

Provider The Provider box lists the code number and name of a patient's assigned provider. If a patient sees a different provider for a visit, the Provider box can be changed to list that provider instead.

TOS TOS stands for "type of service." Medical offices may set up a list of codes to indicate the type of service performed. For example, 1 may indicate an examination, 2 a lab test, and so on. The TOS code is specified in the Procedure/Payment/Adjustment entry for each CPT code.

Diagnosis The Diagnosis 1, 2, 3, and 4 check boxes in the Charge tab correspond to the DIAG 1, 2, 3, and 4 boxes in the main Transaction Entry dialog box. A check mark appears in each Diagnosis box for which a diagnosis was entered in the DIAG 1, 2, 3, 4 boxes. Check marks can be deleted if appropriate. This information is obtained from the Diagnosis tab of the Case folder.

If a patient has several different diagnoses, the diagnosis that is most relevant to the procedure is used. Some insurance carriers do not permit more than one diagnosis per procedure. Diagnoses listed in the Transaction Entry dialog box can be checked or unchecked as needed.

EMC Assignment The 1, 2, and 3 boxes represent up to three insurance policies for transmitting electronic media claims. The 1, 2, and 3 boxes correspond to the insurance carriers listed in the Policy 1, Policy 2, and Policy 3 tabs in a patient's Case dialog box. A check mark indicates that the claim will be transmitted electronically.

SAVING CHARGE TRANSACTIONS

When all the charge information has been entered and checked for accuracy, it needs to be saved. When a transaction is saved, it is added to the list at the bottom of the Transaction Entry dialog box, along with other transactions that have already been entered for the case.

Transactions are saved in MediSoft by clicking one of the buttons grouped vertically at the right side of the Transaction Entry dialog box:

Figure 6-6a
Save/Open button.

Save/Open Clicking the Save/Open button at the top of the group saves the transaction just entered and opens a new tab so that another transaction can be entered (see Figure 6-6a).

Figure 6-6b
Save/Close button.

Save/Close Clicking the Save/Close button (the second button from the top) saves the transaction just entered, closes the tab, and redisplays the main Transaction Entry dialog box (see Figure 6-6b).

Figure 6-6c
Cancel button.

Figure 6-6d
Transaction Documentation button.

Cancel   The Cancel button displays a red "X." This button deletes the transaction data just entered and redisplays the main Transaction Entry dialog box (see Figure 6-6c).

Transaction Documentation   When the Transaction Documentation button located at the bottom of the group is clicked (see Figure 6-6d), the Transaction Documentation dialog box is displayed (see Figure 6-7). This dialog box is used to store notes about a particular transaction. The Transaction Documentation dialog box is optional; it has to be completed only when there is additional information about a particular transaction that needs to be recorded. MediSoft provides several types of transaction documentation. For example, in the Type dropdown list, a variety of choices are listed, such as Diagnostic Report, Operative Note, and Transaction Note (internal use only). After information is entered in the Documentation/Notes box, it is saved by clicking the OK button. The information can be deleted by clicking the Cancel button. A Help button is also available within the Transaction Documentation dialog box.

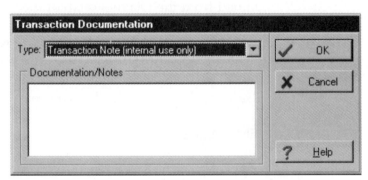

Figure 6-7 **Transaction Documentation dialog box.**

Exercise 6-1

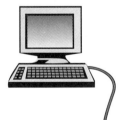

Using Source Document 2, enter a charge transaction for Hiro Tanaka's accident case.

Date: October 4, 2004

1. **Start MediSoft and change the MediSoft Program Date to October 4, 2004, if it is not already set to that date.**

2. **On the Activities menu, click Enter Transactions. The Transaction Entry dialog box is displayed.**

3. **Key *T* in the Chart box and then press Enter to select Hiro Tanaka. Verify that the Accident - back pain case is the active case in the Case box.**

4. **Click the New button. An Information dialog box is diplayed with a message about Tanaka's allergies. Click the OK button to close the box. The Charge tab is displayed.**

5. Verify that the entry in both Dates boxes is 10/4/2004.

6. Accept the default entry in the Document box (0410040000).

7. Key *99202* in the Procedure box to select the procedure code for the service checked off on the superbill. Press Enter.

8. Since there are no modifiers to the procedure code, the Modifiers boxes are left blank.

9. Accept the default entry of 11 in the POS box.

10. Leave the Description box blank.

11. Keep "1" in the Units box.

12. Accept the charge for the procedure that is displayed in the Amount box ($62.00).

13. Accept the information displayed in the Provider box, leave the TOS box blank, and accept the information in the Diagnosis and EMC Assignment boxes.

14. Check your entries for accuracy.

15. Click the Save/Close button to return to the main Transaction Entry dialog box. This is accomplished by clicking the second button from the top in the group of buttons at the right side of the dialog box. An Information box is displayed, stating that a $15 copayment is due for the office visit. You will enter this copayment in Chapter 7, Entering Payments and Adjustments. For now, click the OK button. Notice that the transaction just entered is now listed at the bottom of the dialog box.

Exercise 6-2

Using Source Document 4, enter a charge transaction for Elizabeth Jones' diabetes case.

Date: October 4, 2004

1. If necessary, open the Transaction Entry dialog box.

2. Key *JO* in the Chart box and press Enter to select Elizabeth Jones. Verify that the Diabetes case is the active case in the Case box.

3. Click the New button. The Charge tab is displayed.

4. Accept the default in the Dates boxes (10/4/2004).

5. Accept the default entry in the Document box (0410040000).

6. Key *99213* in the Procedure box to select the procedure code for the services checked off on the superbill. Press Enter

7. Since there are no modifiers to the procedure code, the Modifiers boxes are left blank.

8. Accept the default entry of 11 in the POS box.

9. Leave the Description box blank.

10. Keep "1" in the Units box.

11. Accept the charge for the procedure that is displayed in the Amount box ($39.00).

12. Accept the information displayed in the Provider box; leave the TOS box blank; and accept the information in the Diagnosis and EMC Assignment boxes.

13. Check your entries for accuracy.

14. Click the Save/Close button to return to the main Transaction Entry dialog box. Notice that the transaction just entered is now listed at the bottom of the dialog box.

Exercise 6-3

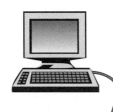

Using Source Document 5, enter the first procedure charge listed for John Fitzwilliams' acute gastric ulcer case.

Date: October 4, 2004

1. If necessary, open the Transaction Entry dialog box.

2. In the Chart box, key *F*. Notice that the chart number for John Fitzwilliams is highlighted on the drop-down list. Press the Enter key. Verify that Acute gastric ulcer is the active case in the Case box.

3. Click the New button. The Charge tab becomes active.

4. Accept the default in the Dates boxes (10/4/2004).

5. Accept the default entry in the Document box (0410040000).

6. Select the procedure code for the services checked off on the superbill. There is more than one procedure. Select the first procedure code (82270). Press Enter.

7. Since a modifier (-90) is listed on the superbill for this procedure, key *90* in the first Modifiers box.

8. Accept the default entry of 11 in the POS box.

9. Leave the Description box blank.

10. Keep "1" in the Units box.

11. Accept the charge for the procedure that is displayed in the Amount box ($19.00).

12. Accept the information displayed in the Provider box; leave the TOS box blank; and accept the information displayed in the Diagnosis and EMC Assignment boxes.

13. Check your entries for accuracy.

14. Click the Save/Open button. This is the first of the four buttons grouped on the right side of the dialog box. An Information box is displayed, stating that a $10 copayment is due for the office visit. You will enter this copayment in Chapter 7, Entering Payments and Adjustments. For now, click the OK button.

Now complete the Charge tab for the second procedure circled on the superbill by completing steps 15 through 26.

15. Accept the default in the Dates boxes.

16. Accept the default entry in the Document box.

17. Select the procedure code for the second service checked off on the superbill (99212). Press Enter.

18. Since there are no modifiers to the procedure code, the Modifiers boxes are left blank.

19. Accept the default entry in the POS box.

20. Leave the Description box blank.

21. Keep "1" in the Units box.

22. Accept the charge for the procedure that is displayed in the Amount box ($28.00).

23. Accept the information displayed in the Provider box; leave the TOS box blank; and accept the information displayed in the Diagnosis and EMC Assignment boxes.

24. Check your entries for accuracy.

25. Click the Save/Close button to return to the main Transaction Entry dialog box. Notice that the two transactions just entered are now listed at the bottom of the dialog box.

26. Close the Transaction Entry dialog box.

EDITING AND DELETING TRANSACTIONS

All transactions entered in MediSoft can be edited within the Transaction Entry dialog box. Double-clicking a particular transaction from the list at the bottom of the Transaction Entry dialog box is the fastest way to edit a transaction in MediSoft. Double-clicking opens the transaction and displays the original Charge, Payment, or Adjustment tab, where information can be changed. After changes are made, the data must be saved.

Transactions can also be deleted from the Transaction Entry dialog box. Clicking the transaction on the list at the bottom of the dialog box highlights the transaction. Once the transaction is highlighted, clicking the right mouse button brings up a shortcut menu. The shortcut menu lists the following commands: Edit Transaction, New Transaction, and Delete Transaction. Clicking Delete Transaction causes a Confirm dialog box to be displayed, asking "Are you sure you want to delete this record?" Clicking the Yes button deletes the transaction; clicking the No button cancels the action.

LOCATING TRANSACTION INFORMATION

Sometimes it is necessary to locate certain patients or cases before editing. MediSoft provides two features within the Transaction Entry dialog box that make it easy to locate transaction information: the Search button and the Briefcase button.

SEARCH BUTTON

The Search button, indicated by a magnifying glass, appears in many MediSoft dialog boxes that contain drop-down lists. In the Transaction Entry dialog box, there is a Search button located next to the Chart and Case boxes. This button is used to locate a particular patient or case. When the Search button next to the Chart box is clicked, the Search dialog box appears (see Figure 6-8). Patients are listed in alphabetical order by chart number. However, the list can also be viewed in a different order by clicking the Sort By drop-down list. The sort options provided are Last Name and Patient ID #2, which is a field that can be used to classify patients according to a criterion set by the practice. When Last Name is selected, MediSoft resorts the list of patients and displays them in alphabetical order by last name. The same is true for Patient ID #2, which can be an alpha or numeric field.

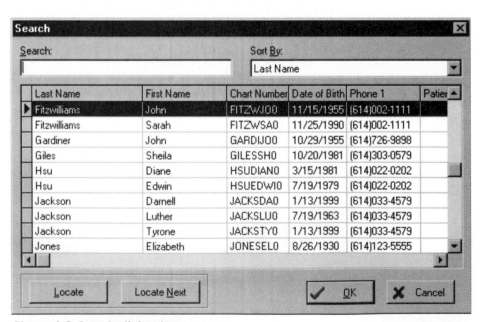

Figure 6-8 **Search dialog box.**

There are two other buttons in the Search dialog box: Locate and Locate Next. The Locate buttons are used to perform searches for specific information, such as assigned provider, employer, date of birth, last payment amount, and so forth. When the Locate button is clicked, the Locate dialog box appears (see Figure 6-9).

The Locate dialog box contains the following boxes:

Field Value   In the Field Value box, the specific characters that match or come close to matching the sought-after information are entered. For example, if someone were searching for a patient with the last name of Silverman, "Silverman" would be entered in the Field Value box. If a search were being conducted for patients of Dr. Singh, "Singh" would be entered.

Search Type   The boxes in the Search Type area of the Locate dialog box provide options that limit the parameters of the search.

Case Sensitive   A check mark in the Case Sensitive box indicates that the items found in the search must match the case of the characters entered in the Field Value box. If this box were checked, a search for "singh" would not return any matches, since the provider's name is in the database as "Singh," with an uppercase "S."

Exact Match   A check mark in the Exact Match box signifies that only information that exactly matches the entry in the Field Value box will be returned in the search.

Partial Match at Beginning   If the Partial Match at Beginning box is checked, the system will return items that match the beginning characters entered in the Field Value box.

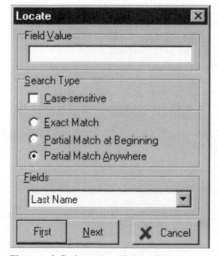

Figure 6-9 **Locate dialog box.**

Partial Match Anywhere   If the Partial Match Anywhere box is checked, the system will return items that match the characters entered in the Field Value box if they appear anywhere in the item. For example, if "son" were entered in the Field Value box, the system would return entries such as "Masterson," "Sonya," and "Wilson's Hardware."

Fields   Searches can be conducted on a variety of different fields of information, including last name, Social Security number, zip code, chart number, assigned provider, and so on. The specific field is selected from the choices in the Fields drop-down list.

First   When the First button is clicked, the system locates the first patient that matches the search criterion and displays that patient's Transaction Entry dialog box. For example, if a search were conducted for patients of Dr. Yan, clicking the First button would display the Transaction Entry dialog box for the first patient (in order of chart numbers) who has Dr. Yan as his or her assigned provider.

Next   When the Next button is clicked, the system locates the next patient who matches the criterion and displays his or her Transaction Entry dialog box.

Cancel   When the Cancel button is clicked, the search is terminated and the Locate dialog box is closed.

The Search and Locate features work the same way in all MediSoft drop-down list boxes.

Exercise 6-4

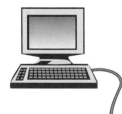

Use the Search feature to locate transactions for a patient.

Date: October 4, 2004

1. Open the Transaction Entry dialog box if it is not already open.

2. Key *A* in the Chart box and press Enter to open Susan Arlen's transactions.

3. Click the Search button next to the Chart box. The Search dialog box is displayed.

4. If it is not already displayed, change the Sort By box to Last Name. Notice that the list is sorted alphabetically by last name.

5. Key *F* in the Search box and watch what happens. The first last name that begins with the letter "F" is highlighted.

6. With John Fitzwilliams highlighted, click the OK button. The Search dialog box closes, and the Transaction Entry dialog box reappears. However, the transactions displayed are now for John Fitzwilliams, not Susan Arlen.

7. Close the Transaction Entry dialog box.

BRIEFCASE BUTTON

Figure 6-10 **Briefcase button.**

The Briefcase button (see Figure 6-10) provides the opportunity to select cases for a particular patient by transaction date, procedure code, and/or amount. This action is accomplished in the Select Case by Transaction Date dialog box (see Figure 6-11). The right side of this dialog box lists all transactions in the system for a particular patient. The left side contains several boxes that can be used to locate transactions that match certain criteria. These boxes are Date From, Procedure Code, and Amount. Any combination of the procedure dates and/or transaction amounts can be entered in their respective boxes.

For example, suppose a billing clerk needs to locate all transactions for procedures completed during an office visit on May 24, 2004. To search for that information, the patient's chart number would be selected in the Chart box, and then the Briefcase button would be clicked. In the Select Case by Transaction Date dialog box, "05242004" would be entered in the Date From box and then the Apply Filter button would be clicked. Instead of listing all transactions for the patient, the right side of the dialog box now lists only those transactions performed on May 24, 2004.

Similarly, a search can be conducted by procedure code or amount. Searches can be conducted using just one of the criteria, or they may include two or three criteria. When the Clear Filter button is clicked, the full list of transactions is displayed again on the right side of the dialog box. Clicking the Select button selects the particular transaction to which the arrow is pointing. The Cancel button closes the dialog box without making any selection.

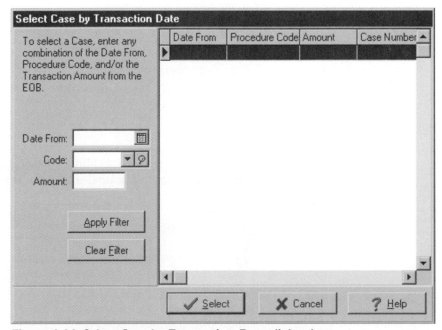

Figure 6-11 **Select Case by Transaction Date dialog box.**

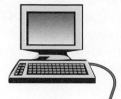

Exercise 6-5

Using the Briefcase button, locate all charges for Paul Ramos that contain procedure code 96900.

Date: October 4, 2004

1. Open the Transaction Entry dialog box.

2. Key *RAMOSP* in the Chart box to select Paul Ramos. Press the Enter key.

3. Click the Briefcase button. The Select Case by Transaction Date dialog box is displayed. Notice that there are several transactions listed for Paul Ramos.

4. In the Code box, key *96900* to select the procedure code. Press Enter.

5. Click the Apply Filter button to begin the search. All transactions that do not match the search criteria are hidden from view; only the transactions that match code 96900 remain visible.

6. Highlight the first transaction, dated 7/12/2004. Press the Select button. The Transaction Entry dialog box appears again, with the case that contains the selected transaction displayed.

7. Close the Transaction Entry dialog box.

ADDITIONAL INFORMATION IN THE TRANSACTION ENTRY DIALOG BOX

The Transaction Entry dialog box also includes other useful information. These data cannot be edited but provide valuable information about a patient and a patient's account. This information is listed in four sections in the Transaction Entry dialog box.

The top right side of the dialog box displays a patient's diagnosis. There are boxes for up to four diagnoses (see Figure 6-12).

DIAG 1, 2, 3, 4   The system copies a patient's diagnosis information from the case file and displays it in the DIAG 1, 2, 3, or 4 box.

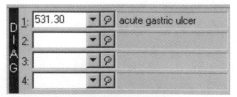

Figure 6-12 **Diagnosis area of Transaction Entry dialog box.**

The section on the left side of the dialog box displays information about the financial responsibilities of the guarantor and the insurance carrier. An estimate of the portion of a bill that will be paid by the insurance carrier(s) is listed, followed by the amount the guarantor is responsible for paying (see Figure 6-13).

Policy 1, Policy 2, Policy 3   A patient's insurance carriers are listed in the Policy 1, Policy 2, and Policy 3 boxes. To the right of the insurance policy is a column labeled "Est. Resp." This is the dollar amount of the estimated responsibility for each insurance carrier.

Guarantor   The system automatically calculates the dollar amount that the guarantor is responsible for paying, after deducting the estimated amount paid by the insurance carrier. This amount is listed in the Guarantor box followed by the guarantor's last name and first name.

Policy Copay   The Policy Copay box lists the amount of a patient's copayment, if applicable.

OA   The Other Arrangements box indicates whether special conditions have been set up for a patient's billing. The system automatically enters information recorded in the Other Arrangements box in the Account tab of the Case dialog box.

Annual Deductible   The Annual Deductible box lists the amount of the patient's annual insurance deductible, if one exists. The YTD (Year-to-Date) box indicates how much of the annual deductible has been meet so far in the current year.

The middle section of the dialog box lists information about the patient's most recent visit and most recent payment (see Figure 6-14).

Last Visit   The Date box within the Last Visit area lists the date of a patient's most recent visit to a particular physician. The Visit box lists the visit series information as entered in the Account tab of the Case dialog box. The Visit box can be edited from within the Transaction Entry dialog box.

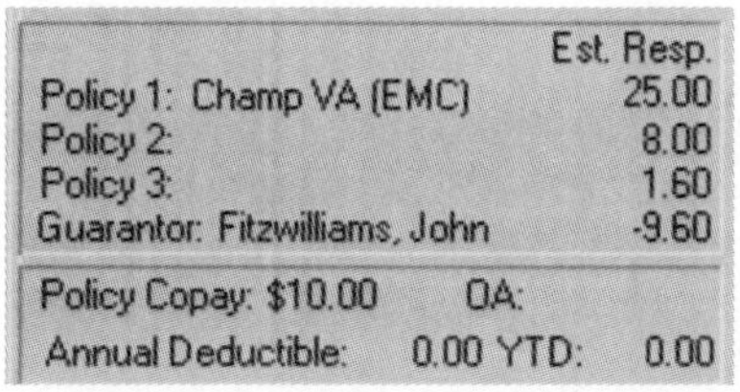

Figure 6-13 **Financial responsibilities area of Transaction Entry dialog box.**

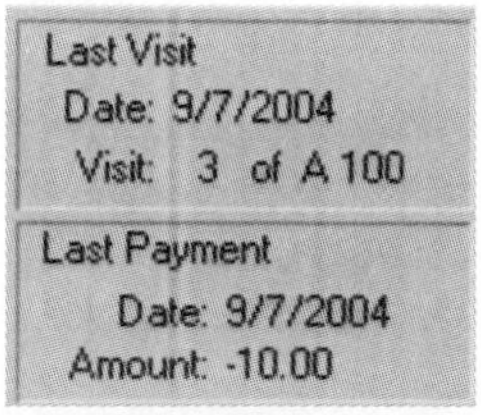

Figure 6-14 **Last Visit and Last Payment area of Transaction Entry dialog box.**

Last Payment   The Last Payment area lists the date (Date box) and the amount of the last payment received (Amount box) on a patient's account.

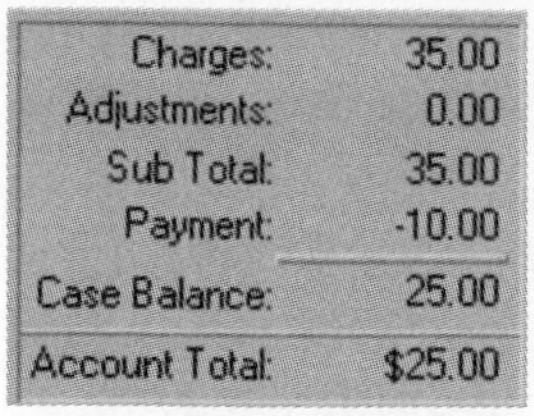

Charges:	35.00
Adjustments:	0.00
Sub Total:	35.00
Payment:	-10.00
Case Balance:	25.00
Account Total:	$25.00

Figure 6-15 Account area of Transaction Entry dialog box.

The right side of the dialog box contains a summary of a patient's account, including charges, adjustments, and payments, for an active case (see Figure 6-15).

Charges   The Charges box lists the total of the charges for a particular case.

Adjustments   The Adjustments box lists the total of the adjustments for this case.

Sub Total   The Sub Total box lists a subtotal of the amounts shown in the Charges and Adjustments boxes. If the amount in the Adjustments box is preceded by a minus sign, that amount is subtracted from the amount in the Charges box.

Payment   The Payment box lists the total payments received to date for this case.

Case Balance   The Case Balance box lists the amount owed for this case .

Account Total   The Account Total box lists the amount owed for a particular patient for all cases, not just the case currently displayed in the Transaction Entry dialog box.

USING TERMINOLOGY

Match the terms on the left with the definitions on the right.

_____ **1.** adjustments

_____ **2.** charges

_____ **3.** modifiers

_____ **4.** MultiLink codes

_____ **5.** payments

a. One- or two-digit codes that add a specific description to a procedure code.

b. Changes to patients' accounts.

c. The amounts billed by a provider for particular services.

d. Monies paid to a medical practice by patients and insurance carriers.

e. Groups of procedure code entries that are related to a single activity.

CHECKING YOUR UNDERSTANDING

Answer the questions below in the space provided.

6. What are the two key pieces of information you must have before entering a procedure charge?

_____

_____

7. List two advantages of using MultiLink codes.

_____

_____

8. Why are charges for copayments made by the patient entered as a separate charge?

_____

_____

9. What is the difference between the Search button and the Briefcase button?

_____

_____

10. What is the Transaction Documentation feature used for?

_____

_____

11. An established patient of Dr. Yan comes in for an emergency visit but cannot get an appointment with Dr. Yan. Instead, she sees Dr. Jessica Rudner. When entering the charge for the visit, how would you indicate that the patient saw Dr. Rudner and not Dr. Yan for that particular office visit?

_____

_____

APPLYING KNOWLEDGE

Answer the questions below in the space provided.

12. After you have entered a charge for procedure code 99212, you realize it should have been 99213. What should you do?

_____

_____

_____

13. The receptionist working at the front desk phones to tell you that Maritza Ramos has just seen the physician and would like to know before she leaves the office what the charges were for her September 8, 2004 office visit. You are in the middle of entering charges from a superbill for another patient. What should you do first? What is your reasoning?

_____

_____

_____

AT THE COMPUTER

Answer the following questions at the computer.

14. Conduct a search for charge transactions for Randall Klein that occurred on September 7, 2004. What are the procedure codes and charges for those transactions?

15. What is the amount of the procedure charge entered on September 10, 2004, for patient Jo Wong?

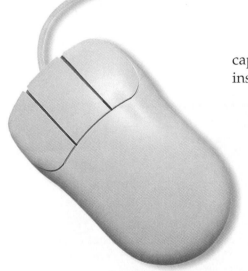

CHAPTER

7

Entering Payments and Adjustments

WHAT YOU NEED TO KNOW

To use this chapter, you need to know how to:
- Start MediSoft, use menus, and enter and edit text.
- Edit information in an existing case.
- Work with chart and case numbers.
- Select patients and cases for transaction entry.

OBJECTIVES

In this chapter, you will learn how to:
- Record and apply payments received from patients.
- Print walkout receipts.
- Record and apply payments received from insurance carriers.

KEY TERMS

capitation payments   patient payments
insurance payments   walkout receipt

ENTERING PAYMENTS IN MEDISOFT

Payments are entered in two different areas of the MediSoft program: the Transaction Entry dialog box, which was introduced in Chapter 6, and the Deposit List dialog box, which will be discussed shortly. Practices may have different preferences for how payments are entered, depending on their billing procedures. In this book, you will be introduced to both methods of payment entry. **Patient payments**—payments made to the practice made directly by the patient or guarantor—will be entered in the Transaction Entry dialog box. This method is convenient for entering patient copayments that are made at the conclusion of an office visit. **Insurance payments**—payments made to the practice on behalf of a patient by an insurance carrier—will be entered in the Deposit List dialog box. The Deposit List feature is more efficient for entering large insurance payments that must be split up and applied to a number of different patients.

ENTERING PATIENT PAYMENTS

Patient payments are entered in the Payment tab of the Transaction Entry dialog box (see Figure 7-1). The Payment tab contains the following boxes:

Date In the Date box, the date when the payment was received is entered. The value in this box defaults to the current date (MediSoft Program Date).

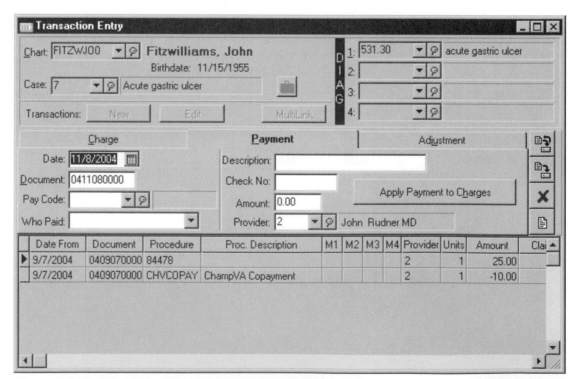

Figure 7-1 **Payment tab of the Transaction Entry dialog box.**

Document Some practices assign document numbers to track charges and payments, others do not. The default entry in this box uses the current date.

Pay Code From the drop-down list in the Pay Code box, the type of payment is selected, such as patient payment, cash; patient payment, check; and various copayment selections.

Who Paid From the drop-down list in the Who Paid box, the party that made the payment is selected. The choices include the patient and the patient's insurance carrier(s).

Description If a payment is made by check, the check number is entered in the Description box. If a payment is not made by check, the Description box can be used to record other information about the payment.

Amount The amount of a payment is entered in the Amount box.

Provider This box lists the name of the provider who treated the patient.

APPLYING AND SAVING PATIENT PAYMENTS

After the Payment tab's boxes have been completed and checked for accuracy, the payment must be applied to charges. This is accomplished by clicking the Apply Payment to Charges button. The Apply Payment to Charges dialog box is then displayed (see Figure 7-2). The dialog box lists information about all unpaid charges for a patient, including the date of the procedure, the document number, the procedure code, the charge, the balance, and the total amount paid. In the top right corner of the dialog box, the amount of payment that has not

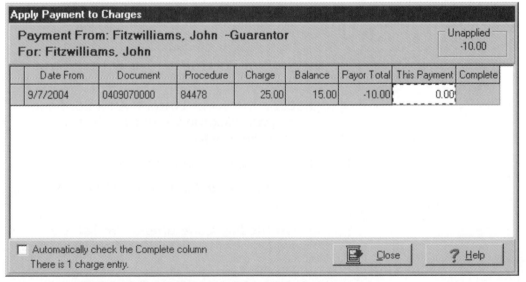

Figure 7-2 **Apply Payment to Charges dialog box.**

yet been applied to charges is listed in the Unapplied box. The cursor appears in the first box of the column labeled "This Payment." Clicking on the zeros in the This Payment box moves the zeros to the top left corner of the box. This indicates that the box is active and ready for entry. The amount of a payment that is to be applied to a charge is entered without a decimal point.

Payments can be applied to more than one charge. For example, suppose that the amount in the Unapplied box is $200 and there are three charges that have not been paid. The $200 payment can be applied to one of the charges or two of the charges, or it can be distributed among the three charges. It is not even necessary to apply the entire payment amount. A balance can remain in the Unapplied box, or the balance can be used to reduce the amount due on another charge.

Clicking the Close button exits the Apply Payment to Charges dialog box, and the Payment tab is again displayed. In the list of transactions at the bottom of the Transaction Entry dialog box, the payment is now listed.

When all the information on a payment has been entered and checked for accuracy, it must be saved. Payment transactions are saved in the manner described earlier for charge transactions. The Transaction Documentation feature is also available in the Payment tab.

Exercise 7-1

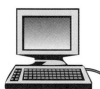

Using Source Document 2, enter the copayment made by Hiro Tanaka for her October 4, 2004, office visit.

Date: October 4, 2004

1. Open the Transaction Entry dialog box.

2. In the Chart box, key *T* and press Enter to select Hiro Tanaka. Verify that Accident - back pain is the active case in the Case box.

3. Click the New button. An Information dialog box is displayed. Click the OK button to close it. Click the Payment tab to make it active.

4. Accept the default entry of 10/4/2004 in the Date box.

5. Accept the default entry of 0410040000 in the Document box.

6. On the Pay Code drop-down list, click OHCCOPAY (the code for OhioCare HMO Copayment) and press Enter.

7. On the Who Paid drop-down list, click Tanaka, Hiro - Guarantor, if she is not already selected.

8. Leave the Description box blank.

9. Key *123* in the Check No. box.

10. If it is not already listed, key *15.00* in the Amount box. Press Tab. Notice that a minus sign appears before the 15.00.

11. Accept the default entry in the Provider box.

12. Click the Apply Payment to Charges button. The Apply Payment to Charges dialog box is displayed.

13. Notice that the amount of this payment (-15.00) is listed in the Unapplied box at the top right of the dialog box.

14. Click the zeros in the This Payment box located on the same line as the charge for October 4, 2004.

15. Key 15 in the This Payment box. Press Tab. The system inserts a decimal point automatically.

16. Click the Close button. The Payment tab is displayed again.

17. Click the Save/Close button to return to the main Transaction Entry dialog box.

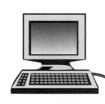

18. Check your entries for accuracy. Notice that the payment just entered is now listed at the bottom of the dialog box. Do not close the Transaction Entry dialog box.

Exercise 7-2

Using Source Document 5, enter the copayment made by John Fitzwilliams for his October 4, 2004, office visit.

Date: October 4, 2004

1. Open the Transaction Entry dialog box.

2. In the Chart box, key *F* and press Enter to select John Fitzwilliams. Verify that Acute gastric ulcer is the active case in the Case box.

3. Click the New button. Make the Payment tab active.

4. Accept the default entry of 10/4/2004 in the Date box.

5. Accept the default entry of 0410040000 in the Document box.

6. On the Pay Code drop-down list, click ChampVA Copayment.

7. On the Who Paid drop-down list, click Fitzwilliams, John - Guarantor, if he is not already selected.

8. Leave the Description box blank.

9. Key *456* in the Check No. box.

10. If it is not already listed, key *10* in the Amount box. Press Tab. Notice that a minus sign appears before the 10.00.

11. Accept the default entry in the Provider box.

12. Click the Apply Payment to Charges button. The Apply Payment to Charges dialog box is displayed.

13. Notice that the amount of this payment (-10.00) is listed in the Unapplied box at the top right of the dialog box.

14. In the list of charges that appears, locate one of the charges for Fitzwilliams' October 4, 2004 office visit. Click the zeros in the This Payment box located on the same line as one of the charges. Notice that the This Payment box is now framed by a dotted box. (In this instance it does not matter which procedure the payment is applied to; both procedures were performed during the office visit to which the payment should be applied.)

15. Key *10* in the This Payment box. Press the Tab key. The system inserts a decimal point automatically.

16. Click the Close button. The Payment tab is displayed again.

17. Click the Save/Close button to return to the main Transaction Entry dialog box.

18. Check your entries for accuracy. Notice that the payment just entered is now listed at the bottom of the dialog box. Do not close the Transaction Entry dialog box.

PRINTING WALKOUT RECEIPTS

walkout receipt *a receipt given to a patient that shows charges, diagnoses, and payments for services*

A **walkout receipt** includes information on the procedures, diagnosis, and charges for a visit. A patient can attach the receipt to an insurance form and submit it directly to his or her carrier. If there is a balance due, the receipt serves as a reminder to the patient of the amount owed.

After a patient payment has been entered in the Transaction Entry dialog box, a walkout receipt is printed and given to the patient before he or she leaves the office. In the Transaction Entry dialog box, a walkout receipt is printed by clicking the Print Receipt button. The Open Report dialog box is displayed, and the available reports are listed under the Report Title heading (see Figure 7-3). Click Walkout Receipt to select the report title, and then click the OK button. MediSoft then asks whether the report is to be previewed on the screen or sent directly to the printer. If the report is to be previewed on screen, it can subsequently be printed directly from the Preview Report window. After the preview/print choice has been made, the Data Selection Questions dialog box is displayed that confirms the patient's chart number and case number, as well as the date of the transaction. The system automatically enters default data in these boxes based on the transaction that is active. Clicking the OK button accepts the default data and sends the report to the printer.

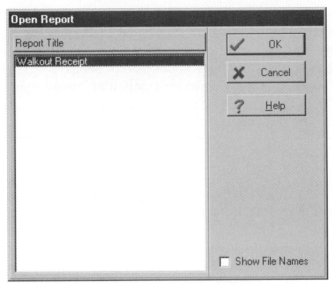

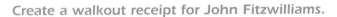

Figure 7-3 **Open Report** dialog box.

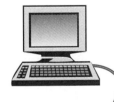

Exercise 7-3

Create a walkout receipt for John Fitzwilliams.

Date: October 4, 2004

1. With the Transaction Entry dialog box open to John Fitzwilliams' acute gastric ulcer case, click the Print Receipt button. The Open Report dialog box is displayed.

2. Verify that Walkout Receipt is highlighted and then click the OK button.

3. In the Print Report Where? dialog box, accept the default selection to preview the report on the screen. Click the Start button.

4. The Data Selection Questions dialog box is displayed. Accept the default entries in the Date From Range boxes and click the OK button. The Preview Report window opens, displaying the walkout receipt.

5. Review the charge and payment entries listed in the top half of the receipt.

6. Scroll down and review the total charges, payments, and adjustments listed at the lower right area of the receipt.

7. Click the Close button to exit the Preview Report window.

8. Close the Transaction Entry dialog box.

ENTERING INSURANCE CARRIER PAYMENTS

Information about payments from insurance carriers is mailed or electronically transmitted to a physician through an electronic remittance advice (RA). A remittance advice lists patients, dates of service, charges, and the amount paid or denied by the insurance carrier. Most RAs also provide an explanation of unpaid charges. Sometimes a paper check is attached to the RA; in other cases the payment is deposited directly in the practice's bank account.

Payment information located on the RA is entered in the Deposit List dialog box. This dialog box is opened by clicking Enter Deposits/ Payments on the Activities menu. The Deposit List dialog box displays a list of all deposits already entered in the program (see Figure 7-4). It contains the following information:

Deposit Date The program displays a default date. The date can be changed by keying over the default date.

Show All Deposits If this box is checked, all payments are displayed—those entered in the Transaction Entry dialog box and those entered in the Deposit List dialog box. If this box is not checked, only payments that were entered in the Deposit List box are visible.

Show Unapplied Only If the Show Unapplied Only box is checked, only payments that have not been fully applied to charge transactions are displayed. If the box is not checked, all payments—both applied and unapplied—are listed.

Sort By The Sort By drop-down list offers two choices for how payment information is listed: the default is sorting payments by description. Payments can also be sorted by the payor name.

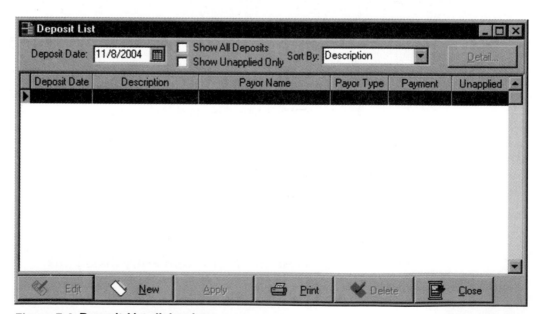

Figure 7-4 **Deposit List dialog box.**

Detail To view detail about a specific deposit, highlight the deposit and click the Detail button.

In the middle section of the window, information is listed for each deposit/payment, including:

Deposit Date lists the date of the deposit or payment.

Description displays whatever was entered in the Description or Check Number box in the Deposit dialog box. The Deposit dialog box is where new payments and deposits are recorded (see Figure 7-5 on page 136). It is accessed by clicking the New button in the Deposit List dialog box.

Payor Name lists the name of the insurance carrier or individual who made the payment.

Payor Type is a classification column; it lists whether the payment is an insurance payment, a patient payment, or a capitation payment. **Capitation payments** are payments made to physicians on a regular basis (such as monthly) as payment for providing services to patients in a managed care insurance plan. In traditional insurance plans, physicians are paid based on the specific procedure they perform, and the number of times the procedure is performed. Under a capitated plan, a flat fee is paid to the physician no matter how many times a patient receives treatment. For example, a physician who is the primary care physician for 50 patients may receive a payment of $2500 per month to provide care for those patients, regardless of whether those patients have been seen by the physician during that month.

Payment lists the amount of the payment.

Unapplied displays the amount of the payment that has not yet been applied to charges.

At the bottom of the Deposit List dialog box are buttons that perform the following actions:

Edit Opens the highlighted payment/deposit for editing.

New Opens the Deposit dialog box, where new payments and deposits are recorded.

Apply Applies payments to specific charge transactions.

Print Sends a command to print the deposit list.

Delete Deletes the highlighted transaction.

Close Exits the Deposit List dialog box.

capitation payments payments made to a physician on a regular basis for providing services to plan members as needed.

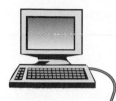

Exercise 7-4

Using Source Document 6, enter the payment received from John Fitzwilliams' insurance carrier for services provided on September 7, 2004.

Date: October 4, 2004

1. Click Enter Deposits/Payments on the Activities menu. The Deposit List dialog box is displayed. Key *10042004* and press the Tab key. Notice that the copayments entered in Exercise 7-1 and 7-2 appear on the deposit list.

2. Click the New button. The Deposit (new) dialog box is displayed (see Figure 7-5).

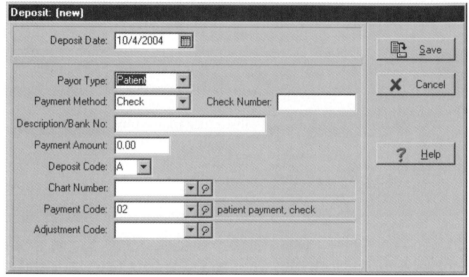

Figure 7-5 **Deposit (new) dialog box.**

3. Verify that the entry in the Deposit Date box is 10/4/2004.

4. Since this is a payment from an insurance carrier, change the selection in the Payor Type box to Insurance.

5. Accept the default entry (Check) in the Payment Method box.

6. Key *214778924* in the Check Number box.

7. The Description/Bank No. field can be left blank.

8. Key 15 in the Payment Amount box.

9. Accept the default entry (A) in the Deposit Code box.

10. Select 5 - ChampVA from the Insurance drop-down list. When an insurance carrier is selected in the Insurance box, MediSoft automatically enters 03–insurance carrier payment in the Payment Code box. Accept this entry.

11. Click the Save button to save the entry and close the Deposit dialog box.

12. The Deposit list box reappears. The insurance payment appears in the list of deposits. Now the payment must be applied to the specific procedure charge to which it is related.

13. With the ChampVA payment entry highlighted, click the Apply button. The Apply Payment/Adjustments to Charges dialog box appears (see Figure 7-6).

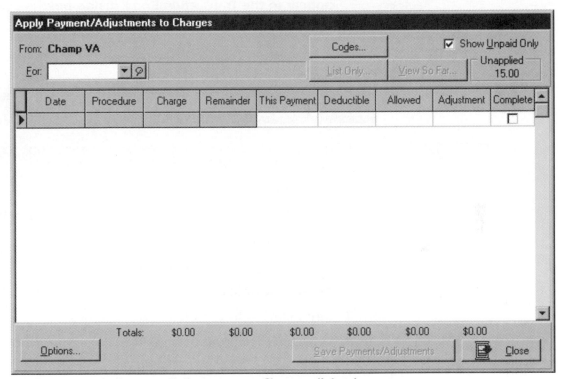

Figure 7-6 **Apply Payment/Adjustments to Charges dialog box.**

14. Key *F* in the For box and press Enter to select John Fitzwilliams, since this payment was for his account. All the charge entries for John Fitzwilliams that have not been paid in full are listed.

15. Since this payment is for the 84478 procedure completed on 09/07/2004, that is the line in which the payment will be applied. Notice that the This Payment box is highlighted.

16. Key *15* in the This Payment box and press Enter. MediSoft automatically places a minus sign before the amount. Notice that once the payment was applied, the Complete box to the right of the dialog box was checked. This indicates that the transaction is complete—the entire amount of the charge has been paid.

17. Click the Save Payments/Adjustments button to save your entry. When you click this button, the dialog box is cleared of the current transactions and is ready for a new transaction.

18. Click the Close button to exit the Apply Payment/Adjustments to Charges dialog box. The Unapplied box for the ChampVA payment on 10/4/2004 is now 0.00.

19. Without closing the Deposit List dialog box, open the Transaction Entry dialog box, select John Fitzwilliams, and verify that an insurance carrier payment appears in the list of transactions. Payments entered in the Deposit List dialog box also appear in the Transaction Entry dialog box.

20. Close the Transaction Entry dialog box.

Exercise 7-5

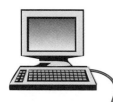

Using Source Document 7, enter a capitation payment from OhioCare HMO for the month of September 2004.

Date: October 4, 2004

1. Click the New button in the Deposit List dialog box.

2. Verify that the entry in the Deposit Date box is 10/4/2004.

3. In the Payor Type box, select Capitation.

4. Accept the default entry of Check in the Payment Method box.

5. Key *78901234* in the Check Number box.

6. Leave the Description/Bank No. box blank.

7. Key *2500* in the Payment Amount box and press Enter.

8. Accept the default entry of A in the Deposit Code box.

9. Click 15–OhioCare HMO in the Insurance drop-down list and press Enter.

10. Click the Save button. The Deposit List window reappears, displaying the payment just entered. Notice that, for this payment, the Unapplied box in the right most column of the dialog box is blank. This is because capitated payments do not need to be applied to individual patients and procedures.

ENTERING INSURANCE PAYMENTS WITH ADJUSTMENTS

Many times insurance carriers do not pay claims in full. Payment may be 80 percent or 50 percent of the charges, or some other amount. Sometimes a change, or an adjustment, needs to be made to a patient's account. When a medical office receives an RA with payments for less than the amount billed, an adjustment transaction must be entered to offset the unpaid charges.

When a payment amount from an insurance carrier is less than the charge amount, MediSoft calculates an estimated adjustment based on data previously entered for that procedure code and insurance carrier. For example, if the charge amount is $60.00 and the insurance carrier paid $48.00 the last time a payment was entered, the program will estimate the adjustment amount to be $12.00 the next time a payment for that procedure code is entered.

Exercise 7-6

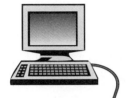

The medical office has just received an RA from Blue Cross/Blue Shield (see Source Document 8). The total amount of the check is $260.80. This amount includes payments for a number of patients. Enter the insurance carrier payment and adjustments for each patient.

Date: November 4, 2004

1. Change the entry in the Deposit Date box to 11/04/2004 and press the Tab key.

2. Click the New button in the Deposit List dialog box.

3. Select Insurance in the Payor Type box.

4. Key *8901* in the Check Number box.

5. Key the RA number, *001234*, in the Description/Bank No. box.

6. Key 260.80 in the Payment Amount box.

7. Accept the default entry in the Deposit Code box.

8. Select 4—Blue Cross/Blue Shield in the Insurance box. MediSoft automatically completes the Payment Code box with 03—insurance carrier payment.

9. Click the Save button.

10. The payment entry appears in the Deposit List dialog box. Notice the amount of $260.80 listed in the Unapplied column for this payment.

Now apply the payment to the specific transaction charges.

11. With the Blue Cross/Blue Shield line highlighted, click the Apply button. The Apply Payment/Adjustments to Charges dialog box is displayed.

12. Key *GI* in the For box to select Sheila Giles, and then press Enter.

13. Locate the charge for procedure code 99213 on 10/29/2004. Key the amount of the payment, *57.60*, in the This Payment box and press Enter. MediSoft automatically checks the Complete box, since Giles only has one insurance carrier (no payment is forthcoming from any other carrier, so the charge is complete).

14. Now enter the payment for the next procedure listed on the RA. Notice that when you click in the This Payment box for the second payment entry, MediSoft calculates the amount still owed on the first procedure charge—the remainder—and displays it in the Remainder column for that charge. In this instance, the remainder is $14.40. Continue entering payments for Giles' other procedures.

15. Click the Save Payments/Adjustments button. The data for Sheila Giles that was visible in the Apply Payment/Adjustments to Charges dialog box is cleared and the dialog box is ready for the next payment or adjustment. Notice also that the amount listed in the Unapplied column for Blue Cross/Blue Shield has been reduced by the amount applied. The unapplied amount is now $84.00.

Now enter the payments for the next patient listed on the RA, Jill Simmons.

16. Key *S* in the For box and press Enter to select Jill Simmons.

17. Enter the payment of 43.20 in the This Payment box for the 99212 charge on 10/29/2004. Press Enter.

18. Enter the other payment for Jill Simmons.

19. Click the Save Payments/Adjustments button. Notice that the amount listed in the Unapplied area of the Apply Payment/Adjustments to Charges dialog box is now 0.00, indicating that the entire payment has been entered.

20. Close the Apply Payment/Adjustments to Charges dialog box.

Exercise 7-7

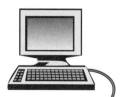

The medical office has just received an RA from East Ohio PPO (see Source Document 9). The total amount of the check is $408.00. This amount includes payments for a number of patients. Enter the insurance carrier payment and adjustments for each patient.

Date: October 4, 2004

1. Change the entry in the Deposit Date box to 10/04/2004 and press the Tab key.

2. Click the New button in the Deposit List dialog box.

3. Select Insurance in the Payor Type box.

4. Key *4567890* in the Check Number box.

5. Key the RA number, *101010*, in the Description/Bank No. box.

6. Key *408.00* in the Payment Amount box and press Tab.

7. Accept the default entry in the Deposit Code box.

8. Select 13—East Ohio PPO in the Insurance box. MediSoft automatically completes the Payment Code box with 03—insurance carrier payment.

9. Click the Save button.

10. The payment entry appears in the Deposit List dialog box. Notice the amount of $408.00 listed in the Unapplied column for this payment.

Now apply the payment to the specific transaction charges.

11. With the East Ohio PPO line highlighted, click the Apply button. The Apply Payment/Adjustments to Charges dialog box is displayed.

12. Key *A* in the For box and press Enter to select Susan Arlen.

13. Locate the charge for procedure code 99212 on 09/06/2004. Key the amount of the payment, *31.00*, in the This Payment box and press Enter. Notice that MediSoft automatically checks the Complete box, since Susan Arlen has only one insurance carrier (there is no payment forthcoming from any other carrier, so the charge is complete).

14. Click the Save Payments/Adjustments button. The data for Susan Arlen that was visible in the Apply Payment/Adjustments to Charges dialog box is cleared and the dialog box is ready for the next payment or adjustment. Notice also that the amount listed in the Unapplied column for East Ohio PPO has been reduced by the amount applied. The unapplied amount is now $377.00.

Now enter the payment for the next patient listed on the RA, Herbert Bell.

15. Key *BE* in the For box and press Enter to select Herbert Bell.

16. Enter the payment of 15.00 in the This Payment box for the 99211 charge on 09/06/2004. Press Enter.

17. Click the Save Payments/Adjustments button.

Apply the insurance carrier payment to Janine Bell's 99213 and 73510 procedures for September 6, 2004.

18. Key *BELLJ* in the For box and press Enter to select Janine Bell.

19. Enter the payment of 47.00 in the This Payment box for the 99213 charge on 09/06/2004. Press Enter.

20. Enter the payment of 103.00 in the This Payment box for the 73510 charge on 09/06/2004. Press Enter.

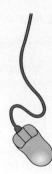

21. Click the Save Payments/Adjustments button.

22. Continue to apply the insurance payments for Jonathan Bell, Samuel Bell, and Sarina Bell using the information on Source Document 9. When you have applied all the payments, the amount in the Unapplied box for the East Ohio PPO payment should be 0.00.

23. Close the Apply Payment/Adjustments to Charges dialog box.

24. Close the Deposit List dialog box.

As you can see, the Deposit List feature makes it possible to enter a number of payment transactions in a short period of time.

USING TERMINOLOGY

Match the terms on the left with the definitions on the right.

_____ **1.** capitation payments

_____ **2.** insurance payments

_____ **3.** patient payments

_____ **4.** walkout receipt

a. Document that is given to a patient at the conclusion of an office visit if a payment has been made.

b. Monies paid to the practice by an insurance carrier for procedure charges.

c. Monies paid to the practice by an insurance carrier for providing treatment to a certain number of patients for a specified period of time.

d. Monies paid to a medical practice by patients in exchange for services.

CHECKING YOUR UNDERSTANDING

Answer the questions below in the space provided.

5. What information does MediSoft use to calculate an estimated adjustment amount?

_____

_____

6. When is it appropriate to print a walkout receipt?

_____

_____

7. Why is it easier to enter large insurance payments in the Deposit List dialog box than in the Transaction Entry dialog box?

_____

_____

8. When all payments on a remittance advice have been successfully entered and applied to charges, what should appear in the Unapplied box in the upper right corner of the Deposit List dialog box?

_____

_____

APPLYING KNOWLEDGE

Answer the questions below in the space provided.

9. After you have entered a payment for $20, you realize it should have been $30. What should you do?

_____

_____

_____

10. The phone rings and it is Randall Klein. He would like to know whether Medicare has paid any of his charges for his September office visit. How would you look up this information in MediSoft?

_____

_____

_____

AT THE COMPUTER

Answer the following questions at the computer.

11. What is the total amount that John Fitzwilliams paid in copayments in September 2004? (*Hint:* Include his daughter Sarah in the calculation.)

12. Today is October 4, 2004. A check for $113.60 arrives from Blue Cross/ Blue Shield as payment for James Smith's facial nerve function studies performed on September 9, 2004. What is the remaining amount of the charge that is James Smith's responsibility to pay? (Do not actually enter the payment in the computer; use MediSoft to look up the necessary information and then calculate the remaining amount.)

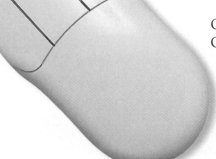

WHAT YOU NEED TO KNOW

To use this chapter, you need to know how to:
◆ Start MediSoft, use menus, and enter and edit text.
◆ Work with chart numbers and codes.

OBJECTIVES

In this chapter, you will learn how to:
◆ Start Office Hours.
◆ View the appointment schedule.
◆ Enter an appointment.
◆ Change or delete an appointment.
◆ Move or copy an appointment.
◆ Search for an existing appointment.
◆ Create a recall list.
◆ Enter a break in a provider's schedule.

KEY TERMS

Office Hours break
Office Hours schedule

INTRODUCTION TO OFFICE HOURS

Appointment scheduling is one of the most important tasks in a medical office. Different medical procedures take different lengths of time, and each appointment must be the right length. On the one hand, physicians want to be able to go from one appointment to another without unnecessary breaks. On the other hand, patients should not be kept waiting more than a few minutes for a physician. Managing and juggling the schedule is usually the job of a medical office assistant working at the front desk. MediSoft provides a special program called Office Hours to handle appointment scheduling.

OVERVIEW OF THE OFFICE HOURS WINDOW

The Office Hours program has its own window (see Figure 8-1) including its own menu bar and toolbar. The Office Hours menu bar lists the menus available: File, Edit, View, Lists, Reports, Tools, and Help (see Figure 8-2). Under the menu bar is a toolbar with shortcut buttons. The functions of Office Hours are accessed by selecting a choice from one of the menus or by clicking a button on the toolbar.

Located just below the menu bar, the toolbar contains a series of buttons that represent the most common activities performed in Office Hours. These buttons are shortcuts for frequently used menu commands. The toolbar displays 14 buttons (see Figure 8-3 and Table 8-1.)

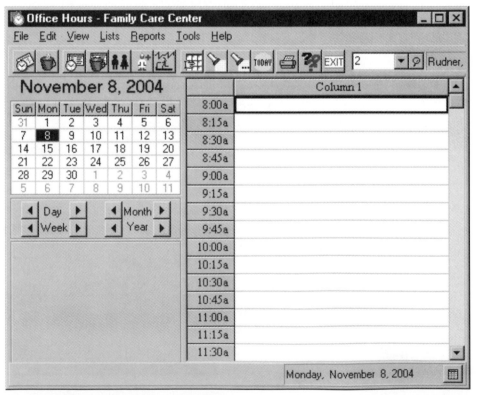

Figure 8-1 **The Office Hours window.**

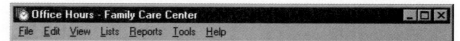

Figure 8-2 **The Office Hours menu bar.**

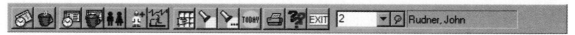

Figure 8-3 **The Office Hours toolbar.**

Table 8-1   Office Hours Toolbar Buttons

Button	Button Name	Associated Function	Activity
	Appointment Entry	New Appointment Entry dialog box	Enter appointments
	Break Entry	New Break Entry dialog box	Enter break
	Appointment List	Appointment List dialog box	Display list of appointments
	Break List	Break List dialog box	Display list of breaks
	Patient List	Patient List dialog box	Displays list of patients
	Provider List	Provider List dialog box	Display list of providers
	Resource List	Resource List dialog box	Display list of resources
	Go to a Date	Go to a Date dialog box	Change calendar to a different date
	Search for Open Time Slot	Find Open Time dialog box	Locate first available time slot
	Search Again	Find Open Time dialog box	Locate next available time slot
	Go to Today		Return calendar to current date
	Print Appointment List		Print appointment list
	Help	Office Hours Help	Display Office Hours Help contents
	Exit Program	Exit	Exit the Office Hours program

The left half of the Office Hours screen displays the current date and a calendar of the current month (see Figure 8-4). The current date is highlighted on the calendar. When a different date is clicked on the calendar, the calendar switches to the new date.

Office Hours schedule *a listing of time slots for a particular day for a specific provider.*

The **Office Hours schedule**, shown in the right half of the screen, is a listing of time slots for a particular day for a specific provider. The provider's name and number is displayed at the top to the right of the shortcut buttons. The provider can be easily changed by clicking the triangle button in the Provider box.

PROGRAM OPTIONS

When Office Hours is installed in a medical practice, it is set up to reflect the needs of that particular practice. Most offices that use MediSoft already have Office Hours set up and running. However, if MediSoft is just being installed, the options to set up the Office Hours program can be found in the Program Options dialog box, which is accessed by clicking Program Options on the Office Hours File menu.

ENTERING AND EXITING OFFICE HOURS

Office Hours can be started from within MediSoft or directly from Windows. To access Office Hours from within MediSoft, Appointment Book is clicked on the Activities menu. Office Hours can also be

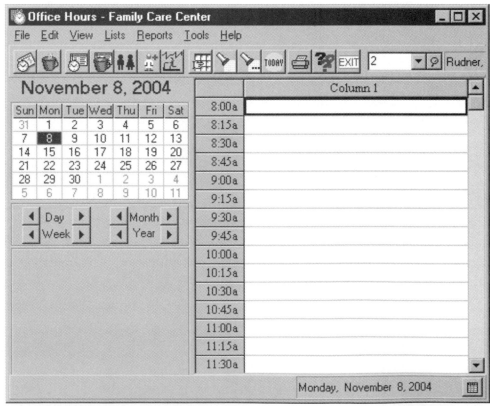

Figure 8-4 **The left side of the Office Hours window displays the current date and a monthly calendar. The right side of the window contains the selected provider's schedule for the current day.**

started by clicking the corresponding shortcut button on the toolbar.

To start Office Hours without entering MediSoft first:

1. Click the Start button on the Windows task bar.

2. Click MediSoft on the Program submenu.

3. Click Office Hours on the MediSoft submenu.

The Office Hours program is closed by clicking Exit on the Office Hours File menu, or by clicking the Exit button on its toolbar. If Office Hours was started from within MediSoft, exiting will return you to MediSoft. If Office Hours was started directly from Windows, clicking Exit will return you to the Windows desktop.

ENTERING APPOINTMENTS

Entering an appointment begins with selecting the provider for whom the appointment is being scheduled. The current provider is listed in the Provider box at the top right of the screen (see Figure 8-5). Clicking the triangle button displays a drop-down list of providers in the system. To choose a different provider, click the name of the provider on the drop-down list.

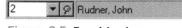

Figure 8-5 **Provider box.**

After the provider is selected, the date of the desired appointment must be chosen. Dates are changed by clicking the Day, Week, Month, and Year right and left arrow buttons located under the calendar (see Figure 8-6). After the provider and date have been selected, patient appointments can be entered.

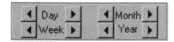

Figure 8-6 **Day, Week, Month, and Year triangle buttons.**

Appointments are entered by clicking the Appointment Entry shortcut button or by double-clicking in a time slot on the schedule. When either of those actions is taken, the New Appointment Entry dialog box is displayed (see Figure 8-7 on page 150). The dialog box contains the following fields:

Chart A patient's chart number is chosen from the Chart drop-down list. To select the desired patient, click on the name and press Enter. If you are setting up an appointment for a new patient who has not been assigned a chart number, skip this box and key the patient's name in the Name box.

Name Once a patient's chart is selected from the Chart drop-down list and the Enter key is pressed, MediSoft displays the patient's name in the Name box. If a patient does not have a chart number, key the patient's name in this box.

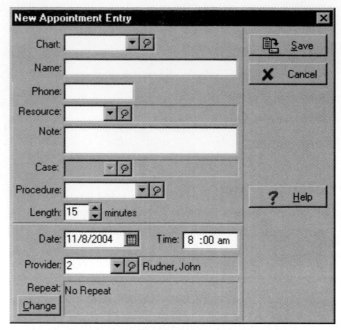

Figure 8-7 **New Appointment Entry dialog box.**

Phone After selecting a patient's chart, that patient's phone number is automatically entered in the Phone box.

Resource This box is used if the practice assigns codes to resources, such as exam rooms or equipment.

Note Any special information about an appointment is entered in the Note box.

Case The case that pertains to the appointment is selected from the drop-down list of cases.

Procedure If the procedure code is known, it is entered in the Procedure Code box by making a selection from the drop-down list of codes or keying the code.

Length The amount of time an appointment will take (in minutes) is entered in the Length box by keying the number of minutes or by using the up and down arrows.

Date The Date box displays the date that is currently displayed on the calendar. If this is not the desired date, it may be changed by keying in a different date or by clicking the calendar button and selecting a date.

Time The Time box displays the appointment time that is currently selected on the schedule. If this is not the desired time, it may be changed by keying in a different time.

Provider The provider who will be treating the patient during this appointment is selected from the drop-down list of providers.

Repeat The Repeat box is used to enter appointments that recur on a regular basis.

After the boxes in the New Appointment Entry dialog box have been completed, clicking the Save button enters the information on the schedule. The patient's name appears in the time slot corresponding to the appointment time. In addition, information about the appointment appears in the lower left corner of the Office Hours window.

LOOKING FOR A FUTURE DATE

Often a patient will need a follow-up appointment at a certain time in the future. For example, suppose a physician has seen a certain patient on a particular day and would like a checkup appointment in three weeks. The most efficient way to search for a future appointment in Office Hours is to use the Go to a Date shortcut button on the toolbar. (This feature can also be accessed on the Edit menu.)

Clicking the Go to a Date shortcut button displays the Go to Date dialog box (see Figure 8-8). Within the dialog box, five boxes offer options for choosing a future date.

Date From This box indicates the current date in the appointment search.

Go __ Days This box is used to locate a date a specific number of days in the future. For example, if a patient needs an appointment 10 days from the current day, "10" would be entered in this box.

Go __ Weeks This box is used when a patient needs an appointment a specific number of weeks in the future, such as six weeks from the current day.

Go __ Months This box is used when a patient needs an appointment a specific number of months in the future, such as three months from the current day.

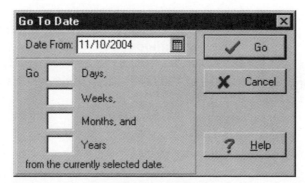

Figure 8-8 **Go To Date dialog box.**

Go __ Years   Similar to the weeks and months options, this box is used when an appointment is needed in one year, or several years in the future.

After a future date option has been selected, clicking the Go button closes the dialog box and begins the search. The system locates the future date and displays the calendar schedule for that date.

Exercise 8-1

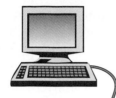

Enter an appointment for Herbert Bell at 2:30 p.m. on Monday, November 15, 2004. The appointment is 15 minutes in length and is with Dr. John Rudner .

1. Start MediSoft. Start Office Hours by clicking the Appointment Book shortcut button on the toolbar.

2. Click 2 - John Rudner on the drop-down list in the Provider box to select John Rudner if he is not already selected.

3. Change the date on the calendar to Monday, November 15, 2004. Use the forward arrow keys to change the month and year, and then click the day in the calendar itself.

4. In the schedule, double-click the 2:30 p.m. time slot. (You will need to use the scroll bar to view 2:30 p.m.) The New Appointment Entry dialog box is displayed.

5. Click Herbert Bell from the list of names on the drop-down list in the Chart box and press Enter. The system automatically fills in a number of boxes in the dialog box, such as the patient's name and phone number.

6. Accept the default entry in the Case box.

7. Notice that the Length box already contains an entry of 15 minutes. This is the default appointment length set up in MediSoft. Since Herbert Bell's appointment is for an annual exam, this entry must be changed to 60 minutes. Key 60 in the Length box or use the up arrow next to the length box to change the appointment length to 60 minutes.

8. Verify the entries in the Date, Time, and Provider boxes and then click the Save button. MediSoft saves the appointment, closes the dialog box, and displays the appointment on the schedule, as well as in the lower left corner of the Office Hours window. Herbert Bell's name is displayed in the 2:30 p.m. time slot on the schedule.

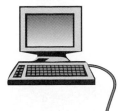

Exercise 8-2

Enter the following appointments with Dr. John Rudner.

1. The first appointment is Monday (November 15, 2004) at 3:30 p.m. for John Fitzwilliams, 30 minutes in length. Verify that "2 Rudner, John" is displayed in the Provider box.

2. In the schedule, double-click the 3:30 p.m. time-slot box.

3. Select John Fitzwilliams on the Chart drop-down list.

4. Press the Enter key. The program automatically completes several boxes in the dialog box.

5. Press the Tab key until the entry in the Length box is highlighted.

6. Key *30* in the Length box or click the up arrow once to change the length to 30 minutes.

7. Click the Save button. Verify that the appointment for John Fitzwilliams appears on the schedule for November 15, 2004, at 3:30 p.m. for a length of 30 minutes.

8. Enter an appointment on Monday, November 15, 2004, at 4:00 p.m. for Leila Patterson, 15 minutes in length.

9. Enter an appointment on Tuesday, November 16, 2004, at 12:15 p.m. for James Smith, 30 minutes in length.

10. To schedule an appointment two weeks after November 16, 2004, for James Smith at 12:15 p.m., 15 minutes in length, click the Go To a Date shortcut button.

11. Key 2 in the Go ____ Weeks box. Click the Go button. The program closes the Go To a Date box and displays the appointment schedule for November 30, 2004.

12. Enter James Smith's appointment.

Exercise 8-3

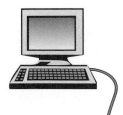

Enter these appointments with Dr. Jessica Rudner.

1. Click Dr. Jessica Rudner from the list of providers in the Provider drop-down list.

2. Enter an appointment for Friday, November 19, 2004, at 2:00 p.m. for Janine Bell, 15 minutes in length.

3. Use Office Hours' Go to a Date feature to schedule an appointment three weeks from November 19, 2004 at 1:15 p.m. for Sarina Bell, 30 minutes in length.

4. Schedule an appointment for Sarah Fitzwilliams one week from November 19, 2004, at 9:00 a.m., 15 minutes in length.

5. Temporarily leave Office Hours by clicking the minimize button in the upper right corner of the window.

Exercise 8-4

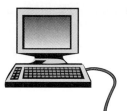

Enter an appointment on Thursday, November 11, 2004, at 9:00 a.m. for John Gardiner, 30 minutes in length. You do not know his provider, so this information must be looked up in MediSoft before you enter the appointment.

1. Go to the Patient List dialog box.

2. Select John Gardiner as the patient.

3. Click the Other Information tab to find out his assigned provider.

4. Click the Office Hours button on the Windows task bar (bottom of screen). Notice that the Patient/Guarantor dialog box is still partially visible underneath the Office Hours window.

5. Select Gardiner's provider in the Provider box in Office Hours.

6. Enter the appointment.

7. Minimize Office Hours.

8. In MediSoft, close the open dialog boxes.

SEARCHING FOR AVAILABLE APPOINTMENT TIME

Often it is necessary to search for available appointment space on a particular day of the week and at a specific time. For example, a patient needs a 30-minute appointment and would like it to be during his lunch hour, which is from 12:00 p.m. to 1:00 p.m. He can get away from the office only on Mondays and Fridays. Office Hours makes it easy to locate an appointment slot that meets these requirements with the Search for Open Time Slot shortcut button.

Exercise 8-5

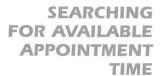

Search for the next available appointment slot beginning November 11, 2004, with Dr. Yan, on a Thursday or Tuesday, between the hours of 11:00 a.m. and 2:00 p.m.

1. Click the Office Hours button on the Windows taskbar. Verify that Dr. Katherine Yan is displayed next to the Provider box.

2. On the Edit menu, click Find Open Time, or click the Search for Open Time Slot shortcut button. The Find Open Time dialog box is displayed (see Figure 8-9).

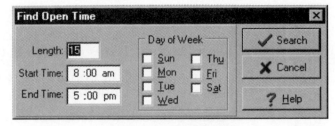

Figure 8-9 **Find Open Time dialog box.**

3. Key *30* in the Length box. Press the Tab key.

4. Key *11* in the Start Time box.

5. Key *2* in the End Time box.

6. To search for an appointment on Tuesday or Thursday, click the Tuesday and Thursday boxes in the Day of Week area of the dialog box.

7. Click the Search button to begin looking for an appointment slot. MediSoft closes the dialog box and locates the first available time slot that meets these specifications. The time slot is outlined on the schedule.

8. Double-click the selected time slot. Click Maritza Ramos on the drop-down list in the Name box.

9. Press the Tab key until the cursor is in the Length box.

10. Key *30* and press the Tab key.

11. Click the Save button.

12. Verify that the appointment has been entered by looking at the schedule.

Exercise 8-6

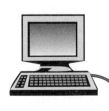

Schedule Randall Klein for a 30-minute appointment with Dr. John Rudner on November 15, 2004. Mr. Klein is available only between 3:00 p.m. and 5:00 p.m.

1. Click the desired provider in the Provider box.

2. Change the calendar to November 15, 2004.

3. Click Find Open Time on the Edit menu to display the Find Open Time dialog box.

4. In the Length box, highlight the number already entered and key *30*. Press the Tab key to move the cursor to the Start Time box.

5. Key *3* in the Start Time box. Press Tab twice to move the cursor to the am selection.

6. Key *p* to change am to pm. Press Tab to move to the End Time box.

7. Key *5* in the End Time box.

8. In the Day of Week boxes, select Monday. Click the Tuesday and Thursday boxes to deselect those days.

9. Click the Search button. The first available slot that meets the requirements is outlined on the schedule.

10. Double-click in the time slot to open the New Appointment Entry dialog box.

11. Click Randall Klein from the drop-down list in the Chart box. Press tab several times to move the cursor to the Length box.

12. Key *30* in the Length box, and press the Tab key.

13. Click the Save button. The dialog box closes and Randall Klein's appointment appears on the schedule.

ENTERING APPOINTMENTS FOR NEW PATIENTS

When a new patient phones the office for an appointment, the appointment can be scheduled in Office Hours before the patient information is entered in MediSoft. However, while the prospective patient is still on the phone, most offices obtain basic data and enter it in the appropriate MediSoft dialog boxes (Patient/Guarantor and Case).

Exercise 8-7

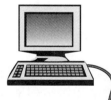

Schedule Lisa Green, a new patient, for a 45-minute appointment with Dr. John Rudner on November 15, 2004, at 1:45 p.m.

1. Verify that November 15, 2004, is displayed on the schedule and that Dr. John Rudner is selected as the provider.

2. Double-click the 1:45 p.m. time slot

3. Click in the Name box and key Lisa Green. Press the Tab key to move the cursor to the Phone box.

4. Key *6145553604* in the Phone box and press Tab three times. The cursor should be in the Procedure box.

5. Key *99203* to select the procedure. Press Tab once.

6. Key *45* in the Length box.

7. Click the Save button. The appointment is displayed on the November 15, 2004 schedule.

BOOKING REPEATED APPOINTMENTS

Some patients require appointments on a repeated basis, such as every Thursday for eight weeks. Repeated appointments are also set up in the New Appointment Entry dialog box. The Repeat feature is located at the bottom of the dialog box. When the Change button is clicked, the Repeat Change dialog box is displayed. The Repeat Change dialog box provides a number of choices for setting up repeating appointments (see Figure 8-10).

The left side of the dialog box contains information about the frequency of the appointments. The default is set to None. Other options include Daily, Weekly, Monthly, and Yearly. When an option other than None is selected, the center section of the dialog box changes and displays additional options for setting up the appointments (see Figure 8-11).

In the center section, an option is provided to indicate how often the appointments should be scheduled, such as every 1 week. Below that there is an option to indicate the day of the week on which the appointment should be scheduled. Finally, there is a box to indicate when the repeating appointments should stop. When all the information has been entered, clicking the OK button closes the Repeat Change dialog box and the New Appointment Entry dialog box is once again visible. Clicking the Save button enters the repeating appointments on the schedule.

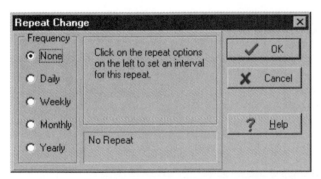

Figure 8-10 **Repeat Change dialog box when None is selected.**

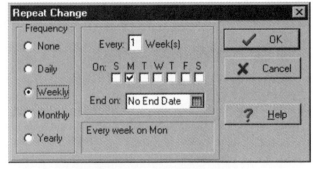

Figure 8-11 **Repeat Change dialog box when an option other than None is selected.**

Exercise 8-8

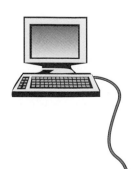

Schedule Li Y. Wong for a 15-minute appointment with Dr. Katherine Yan, once a week for six weeks. Mrs. Wong has requested that the appointments be at the same time every week, preferably in the early morning, beginning with Wednesday, November 17, 2004.

1. Click the desired provider on the Provider drop-down list.

2. Change the schedule to November 17, 2004.

3. Double-click in the 8:00 a.m. time slot. The New Appointment Entry dialog box is displayed.

4. Select Li Y. Wong from the Chart drop-down list. Press the Tab key.

5. Confirm that the entry in the Length box is 15 minutes.

6. Click the Change button to schedule the repeating appointments.

7. In the Frequency column, select Weekly.

8. Accept the default entry of 1 in the Every __ Weeks box.

9. Accept the default entry of W to accept Wednesday as the day of the week.

10. Click the small calendar icon to the right of the End on box. A calendar pops up. Count six weeks from November 17, 2004. (Note: You will have to click the drop-down triangle next to November and change the calendar to display November 17, 2004.) When you find the sixth Wednesday (counting November 17 as the first week), double-click in the calendar box for that day. 12/22/2004 appears in the End on box.

11. Click the OK button. Notice that "Every week on Wed" is displayed in the Repeat area of the New Appointment Entry dialog box.

12. Click the Save button to enter the appointments. Notice that "Occurs every week on Wed" appears in the lower left corner of the Office Hours window.

13. Go to December 22, 2004, to verify that Mrs. Wong is scheduled for an appointment at 8:00 a.m.

14. Go to December 29, 2004, and confirm that Mrs. Wong is not scheduled. This is the seventh week, and her repeating appointments were only scheduled for six weeks, so no appointment should appear on December 29, 2004.

CHANGING OR DELETING APPOINTMENTS

Very often it is necessary to change a patient's appointment or cancel an appointment. Changing an appointment is accomplished with the Cut and Paste commands on the Office Hours Edit menu.

The following steps are used to reschedule an appointment:

1. Locate the appointment that needs to be changed. Make sure the appointment slot is visible on the schedule.

2. Click on the existing time-slot box. A black border surrounds the slot to indicate that it is selected.

3. Click Cut on the Edit menu. The appointment disappears from the schedule.

4. Click the date on the calendar when the appointment is to be rescheduled.

5. Click the desired time-slot box on the schedule. The slot becomes active.

6. Click Paste on the Edit menu. The patient's name appears in the new time-slot box.

The following steps are used to cancel an appointment without re-scheduling:

1. Locate the appointment on the schedule.

2. Click the time-slot box to select the appointment.

3. Click Cut on the Edit menu. The appointment disappears from the schedule.

TIP> Instead of using the Cut and Paste commands to change or delete an appointment, select the appointment and press the right mouse button. A shortcut menu appears with several options, including Cut, Copy, and Delete.

Exercise 8-9

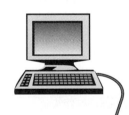

Change Janine Bell's and John Gardiner's appointments.

1. Click Jessica Rudner on the Provider box drop-down list.

2. Go to Friday, November 19, 2004, on the calendar.

3. Locate Janine Bell's 2:00 p.m. appointment on the schedule. Click the 2:00 p.m. time-slot box.

4. Click Cut on the Edit menu. Janine Bell's appointment is removed from the 2:00 p.m. time-slot box. (You may also use the right mouse click shortcut)

5. Click the 3:00 p.m. time-slot box.

6. Click Paste on the Edit menu. Janine Bell's name is displayed in the 3:00 p.m. time-slot box.

7. Click Katherine Yan on the Provider drop-down list.

8. Go to Thursday, November 11, 2004, on the calendar.

9. Locate John Gardiner's 9:00 a.m. appointment. Remove his appointment from the 9:00 a.m. time slot.

10. **Go to Friday, November 19, 2004, on the calendar.**

11. **Enter John Gardiner's appointment in the 9:15 a.m. time slot.**

12. **Exit Office Hours.**

CREATING A RECALL LIST

Medical offices frequently must keep track of patients who need to return for future appointments. Some offices schedule future appointments when the patient is leaving the office. For example, if a patient has just seen a physician and needs to return for a follow-up appointment in six weeks, the appointment is usually made before the patient leaves the office. However, when the appointment is needed some time farther in the future, such as one year later, it is not always practical to set up the appointment. It is difficult for the patient and for the physician to know their schedules a year in advance. For this reason, many offices keep a list of patients who need to be contacted for future appointments.

In MediSoft, a recall list can be created and maintained by clicking Patient Recall on the Lists menu. Patients can also be added to the recall list by clicking the Patient Recall Entry shortcut button on the toolbar. When Patient Recall is selected from the Lists menu, the Patient Recall List dialog box is displayed (see Figure 8-12). This dialog box organizes the recall information in a column format. The scroll bar is used to display the last three columns on the right.

◆ **Date of Recall** Lists the date the recall is scheduled.

◆ **Name** Displays the patient's name.

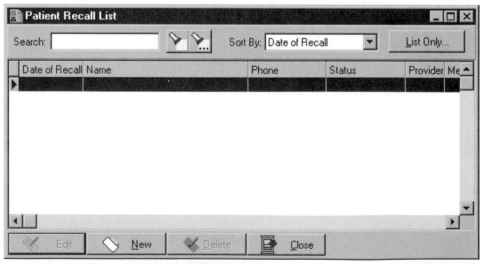

Figure 8-12 *Patient Recall List dialog box.*

- **Phone** Lists the patient's phone number, making it easy to call patients for appointments without having to look up phone numbers in another dialog box.

- **Status** Indicates the patient's recall status: Call, Call Again, Appointment Set, No appointment.

- **Provider** Displays the provider code for the patient's provider.

- **Message** Displays the entry made in the Message box of the Patient Recall dialog box.

- **Extension** Lists the patient's phone extension.

- **Chart Number** Displays the patient's chart number.

- **Procedure Code** Lists the procedure code for the procedure for which the patient is being recalled.

The Patient Recall List dialog box contains the following boxes:

Search The Search box is used to locate a specific patient on the recall list. Entering the first few letters or numbers in the Search box displays the selection that is the closest match to the search criteria.

Sort By The choices in the Sort By box determine whether patients are listed in the dialog box by Date of Recall, Chart Number, or Provider. The default entry is Date of Recall.

The Patient Recall List dialog box also contains these buttons: List Only, Edit, New, Delete, and Close.

List Only The List Only button is used to temporarily select the list of patients who are on the recall list in the Patient Recall List dialog box. When the List Only button is clicked, the List Only Recalls That Match dialog box is displayed with five radio buttons that correspond to the patient's recall status: Call, Call Again, Appointment Set, No Appointment, and All. The latter is used to select all patients regardless of recall status. For example, if the Call radio button is selected, the dialog box lists only those patients who require phone calls. To apply the option selected, the OK button is clicked and the revised list of patients is displayed in the Patient Recall List dialog box. Data on the other patients are not deleted, just temporarily hidden from view. To see the full list of patients, reenter the List Only Recalls That Match dialog box by clicking the List Only button, click the All radio button, and click the OK button.

Edit Clicking the Edit button displays the Patient Recall dialog box for the patient whose entry is highlighted. The information on the patient can then be edited by making different selections in the boxes.

New   Clicking the New button displays an empty Patient Recall dialog box, in which data on a new recall patient can be entered.

Delete   Clicking the Delete button deletes from the patient recall list data on the patient whose entry is highlighted.

Close   The Close button is used to exit the Patient Recall List dialog box.

ADDING A PATIENT TO THE RECALL LIST   Patients are added to the recall list by clicking the New button in the Patient Recall List dialog box or by clicking the Patient Recall Entry shortcut button. When either of these actions is performed, the Patient Recall dialog box is displayed (see Figure 8-13). The Patient Recall dialog box contains the following boxes:

Recall Date   The date a patient needs to return to see a physician is entered in the Recall Date box.

Provider   A patient's provider is selected from the drop-down list.

Chart   A patient's chart number is selected from the drop-down list, or the first few letters of a patient's chart number are entered in the Chart box.

Name, Phone, Extension   After a chart number is entered, the system automatically completes the Name, Phone, and Extension boxes.

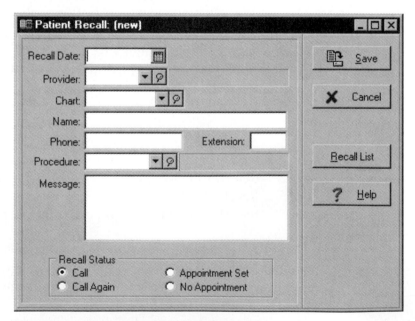

Figure 8-13 **Patient Recall (new) dialog box.**

Procedure   If the procedure for which a patient is returning is known, it is entered in the Procedure box in one of two ways. The procedure code can be selected from the drop-down list, or the first few numbers can be entered and the drop-down list will display the entry that most closely matches the entered numbers. This is especially valuable in practices in which there are hundreds of procedure codes, because it eliminates the need to scroll through several hundred codes to locate the desired one.

Message   The Message box is used to record any special notes, reminders, or instructions about a patient and his or her appointment.

Recall Status   The choices in the Recall Status box are used to indicate the action that needs to be taken. They include:

Call   The Call button is used when a patient needs to be telephoned about a future appointment.

Call Again   The Call Again button is used when a patient has been called once, but contact was not made and an additional call is necessary.

Appointment Set   The Appointment Set button is used when a patient has an appointment already scheduled.

No Appointment   The No Appointment button is used when a patient has been contacted for an appointment but has declined for some reason.

After the information has been entered in the dialog box, clicking the Save button saves the data and adds the patient to the recall list. In addition to the Save button, the Patient Recall dialog box contains these buttons: Cancel, Recall List, and Help. The Cancel button exits the dialog box without saving the data entered. The Recall List button in the Patient Recall dialog box is used to display the Patient Recall List dialog box. The Help button displays MediSoft's online help for the Patient Recall dialog box.

Exercise 8-10

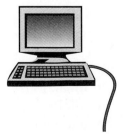

John Fitzwilliams needs to receive a phone call one year from November 15, 2004, to set up an appointment for Procedure 99396, established patient, 40–64 years, periodic preventive medicine. Add John Fitzwilliams to the recall list.

1. **Click the Patient Recall Entry shortcut button. The Patient Recall dialog box is displayed.**

2. **In the Recall Date box, enter November 15, 2005.**

3. Determine which physician is John Fitzwilliams's provider. (Look in the Patient/Guarantor dialog box for this information.)

4. Click John Fitzwilliams' provider on the drop-down list in the Provider box.

5. Enter John Fitzwilliams' chart number in the Chart box by keying the first few letters of his chart number. Notice that the system automatically completes the Phone box. (The Extension box would also be completed if there were an extension).

6. Enter the procedure code in the Procedure box by keying *99396* (established patient, 40-64 years, periodic preventive medicine).

7. In the Message box, key *Was changing jobs; ask about new insurance coverage.*

8. Verify that the Call radio button in the Recall Status box is selected.

9. Click the Save button to save the entry.

10. Click Patient Recall on the Lists menu.

11. Verify that the entry for John Fitzwilliams has been added to the recall list.

12. Close the Patient Recall List dialog box.

CREATING BREAKS

Office Hours break a block of time when a physician is unavailable for appointments with patients.

Office Hours provides features for inserting standard breaks in providers' schedules. The **Office Hours break** is a block of time when a physician is unavailable for appointments with patients. Some examples of breaks include Lunch, Meeting, Personal, Emergency, Break, Vacation, Seminar, Holiday, Trip, and Surgery. In Office Hours, breaks can be created one at a time or on a recurring basis for all providers. One-time breaks, such as those for a vacation, are obviously set up for an individual provider. Other breaks, such as staff meetings, can be entered once for multiple providers.

Often breaks need to be inserted into a provider's schedule when he or she is not available for appointments with patients. For example, if a physician will be in surgery on Thursday from 9 a.m. until 12:00 p.m., that time period must be marked as unavailable on his or her schedule.

To set up a break for a current provider (that is, the provider listed in the Office Hours Provider box), click the Break Entry shortcut button. This action causes the New Break Entry dialog box to appear (see Figure 8-14). The dialog box contains the following options:

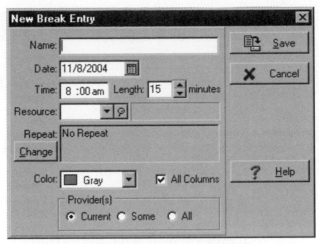

Figure 8-14 **New Break Entry dialog box.**

Name The name field is used to store a name or description of the break.

Date The date field displays the current date on the Office Hours calendar. If this is not the correct date for the break entry, a different date can be entered.

Time The starting time of the break is entered in this box.

Length This box indicates the length of the break in minutes (from 0 to 720).

Resource The drop-down list entries in the Resource box display different types of breaks already set up in Office Hours.

Change The Change button next to the Repeat box is used to enter breaks that recur at a regular interval.

Color By selecting a different color from the drop-down list, the color of the break time slot in the schedule can be changed.

Provider(s) The Provider(s) buttons are used to indicate whether the break is to be set for the current provider (the provider that is selected in the Provider box in Office Hours), some providers, or all providers. If some is selected, a Provider Selection dialog box will be displayed when the Save button is clicked. The appropriate providers can then be selected.

When all the information has been entered, clicking the Save button closes the dialog box and enters the break(s) in MediSoft.

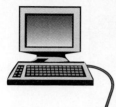

Exercise 8-11

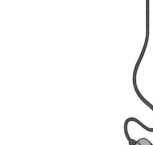

Dr. Jessica Rudner will be away at a seminar from Monday, December 13, 2004, to Wednesday, December 15, 2004. Enter this as a break on her schedule.

1. Start Office Hours.

2. Select Jessica Rudner from the Provider drop-down list.

3. Change the date on the calendar to December 13, 2004.

4. Click the Break Entry shortcut button. The Edit Break dialog box appears.

5. Key *Seminar* over the existing entry in the Name box and press Tab twice to go to the Time box.

6. If it is not already displayed, change the entry in the Time box to 8:00 am. Press Tab until you reach the Length box.

7. Key *540* in the Length box to indicate that the break is all day (9 hours). Press Tab once.

8. Select Seminar Break from the choices on the Resource drop-down list.

9. Press the Change button (to repeat the break for two additional days). The Repeat Change dialog box is displayed.

10. Click the Daily button in the Frequency column. The center of the dialog box changes to display more options.

11. Accept the default entry of 1 in the Every __ Day(s) box, since the break occurs every day for a period of three days.

12. Key *12152004* in the End on box.

13. Click the OK button. You are returned to the Edit Break dialog box.

14. Click the Save button to enter the break in Office Hours. Notice that December 13, 2004, has been filled in on the calendar and the word "Seminar" appears next to the 8:00 a.m. time slot.

15. Change the calendar to December 14 and 15, 2004, to verify that the break has been entered correctly.

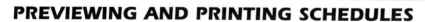

PREVIEWING AND PRINTING SCHEDULES

In most medical offices, providers' schedules are printed on a daily basis. To view a list of all appointments for a provider for a given day, click Appointment List from the Reports menu. The report can be previewed on-screen or sent directly to the printer. If the preview option is selected, the appointment list is displayed in a preview window (see Figure 8-15). Various buttons are used to view the schedule at different sizes, to move from page to page, to print the schedule, and to save the schedule as a file. Clicking the Close button closes the preview window.

The schedule can also be printed by clicking the Print Appointment List shortcut button, without using the Preview option. (Office Hours prints the schedule for the provider who is listed in the Provider box. To print the schedule of a different provider, change the entry in the Provider box before printing the schedule.)

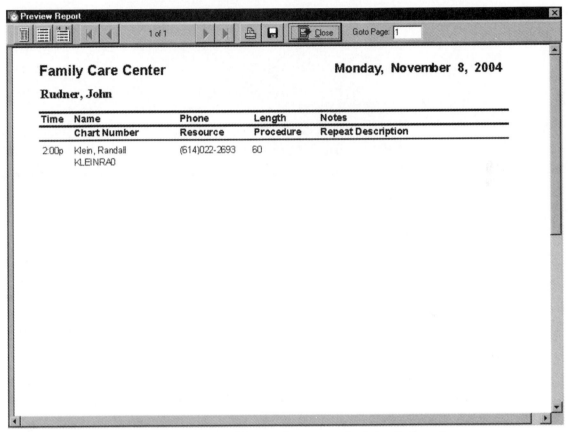

Figure 8-15 **Preview Report window with appointment schedule displayed.**

Exercise 8-12

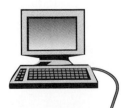

Print Dr. John Rudner's schedule for November 15, 2004.

1. Select Dr. John Rudner as the provider.

2. Go to Monday, November 15, 2004, on the calendar.

3. Click Appointment List on the Office Hours Reports menu. The Print Report dialog box appears.

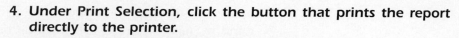

4. Under Print Selection, click the button that prints the report directly to the printer.

5. Under Report Type, click Detail.

6. Click the Start button. The Print dialog box appears.

7. Click OK to print the report.

8. Close Office Hours.

9. Exit MediSoft.

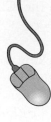

CHAPTER REVIEW

USING TERMINOLOGY

Define the terms below as they apply to Office Hours.

1. Office Hours schedule

_____

_____

2. Office Hours break

_____

_____

CHECKING YOUR UNDERSTANDING

Answer the questions below in the space provided.

3. What are the different ways of starting Office Hours?

_____

_____

4. How do you display the schedule for a specific date?

_____

_____

5. If the calendar shows October 6, how do you move to November 6?

_____

_____

6. How do you display the schedule for a specific provider?

_____

_____

7. How is an appointment deleted?

_____

_____

8. What are two methods that can be used to move an appointment from one time slot to another?

_____

_____

9. Suppose your office has set up Office Hours so that the default appointment length is 15 minutes. If you need to make a one-hour appointment for a patient, in what box do you change 15 to 60?

_____

_____

APPLYING KNOWLEDGE

Answer the questions below in the space provided.

10. After you entered a personal break for Dr. Katherine Yan on February 24, she tells you that she gave you the wrong date. The break should be February 25. How do you correct the schedule?

_____

_____

11. A patient calls to request an appointment on a specific day next week. You determine that the appointment is for a routine checkup, not an emergency. What steps should you follow to schedule the appointment?

_____

_____

AT THE COMPUTER

Answer the following questions at the computer.

12. Dr. Katherine Yan asks you to find out when Sarah Fitzwilliams is coming in for her next appointment. Locate the appointment in Office Hours.

13. Today is November 15, 2004. Samuel Bell needs to be scheduled as soon as possible for a 30-minute appointment with Dr. John Rudner, between 10:00 a.m. and 12:00 p.m. When is the next available time slot that meets these requirements? How did you locate the open slot?

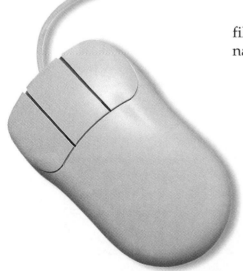

9 Using Claim Management

WHAT YOU NEED TO KNOW

To use this chapter, you need to know how to:
◆ Start MediSoft, use menus, and enter and edit text.
◆ Work with chart numbers and codes.

OBJECTIVES

In this chapter, you will learn how to:
◆ Create electronic claims.
◆ Review claims for errors and omissions.
◆ Review an audit/edit report.

KEY TERMS

filter
navigator buttons

CREATING CLAIMS

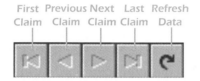

Figure 9-1 **Claim Management shortcut button.**

navigator buttons *buttons that simplify the task of moving from one entry to another.*

First Previous Next Last Refresh
Claim Claim Claim Claim Data

Figure 9-3 **Navigator buttons.**

CREATE CLAIMS DIALOG BOX

filter *a condition that data must meet to be included in the selection of data.*

Within the Claim Management area of MediSoft, insurance claims are created, edited, and submitted for payment. Claims are created from transactions previously entered in MediSoft. After claims are created, they can either be printed and mailed or transmitted electronically. The Claim Management dialog box is displayed by clicking Claim Management on the Activities menu or by clicking the Claim Management shortcut button on the toolbar (see Figure 9-1). This dialog box (see Figure 9-2) lists all claims that have already been created. In this dialog box, several actions can be performed: existing claims can be reviewed and edited, new claims can be created, the status of existing claims can be changed, and claims can be printed or submitted electronically.

The Claim Management dialog box contains five **navigator buttons** that simplify the task of moving from one entry to another (see Figure 9-3). The First Claim button selects the first claim in the list and makes it active. The Previous Claim button reactivates the claim that was most recently active. The Next Claim button makes the next claim in the list active. The Last Claim button makes the last claim in the list active. The Refresh Data button is used to restore data when necessary.

Claims are created in the Create Claims dialog box. The Create Claims dialog box (see Figure 9-4) is accessed by clicking the Create Claims button in the Claim Management dialog box. This dialog box provides several filters to customize the creation of claims. A **filter** is a condition that data must meet to be included in the selection of data. For example, claims can be created for services performed between the first and the fifteenth of the month. If this were the case, the filter would be the condition that services must have been performed between the first

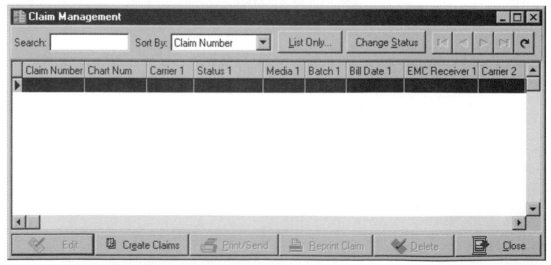

Figure 9-2 **Claim Management dialog box.**

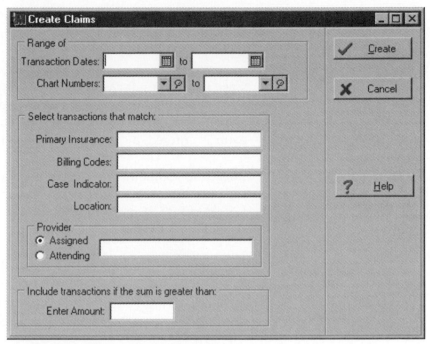

Figure 9-4 **Create Claims dialog box.**

and fifteenth of the month. Transactions that meet this criterion would be included in the selection; transactions that do not fall within that date range would not be included. Filters can be used to create claims for a specific patient, for a specific insurance carrier, for transactions that exceed a certain dollar amount, and so on. The following filters can be applied within the Create Claims dialog box.

Range of The options in this section of the dialog box provide filters for establishing the starting and ending dates as well as the starting and ending chart numbers for the claims that will be created.

Transaction Dates The Transaction Dates boxes are used to specify the starting and ending dates for which claims will be created. If the boxes are left blank, transactions for all dates will be included.

Chart Numbers In the Chart Numbers boxes, the starting and ending chart numbers for which claims will be created are entered. If the boxes are left blank, all chart numbers will be included.

Select Transactions That Match The options in this section of the dialog box provide filters for matching the exact primary insurance carrier(s), billing code(s), case indicator(s), and location(s).

Primary Insurance The carrier code for the insurance company is entered in the Primary Insurance box. If claims are being sent to a clearinghouse, more than one insurance carrier code can be entered. When more than one code is entered, a comma must be placed between the codes. If claims are being sent directly to the carrier, only that carrier's code is entered.

Billing Codes The billing code is entered in the Billing Codes box. If more than one code is entered, a comma must be placed between the codes.

Case Indicator If case indicators are used to classify patients (such as by type of illness for workers' compensation cases), the case indicator can be listed in the Case Indicator box. If more than one indicator is entered, a comma must be placed between each one.

Location Sometimes a sort is needed by location, such as all procedures done at a hospital. The location code is entered in the Location box. If more than one code is entered, a comma must be placed between the codes.

Provider The radio buttons in the Provider box indicate whether the provider is the assigned or attending provider. In the box to the right of the radio buttons, the provider code is entered. If more than one code is entered, a comma must be placed between the codes.

Include Transactions if the Sum Is Greater Than The dollar amount entered in this box is the minimum total amount required for a case before a claim can be created.

Any box that is not filled in will default to include all data, and claims with any entry in that box will be included. When all necessary information has been entered, clicking the Create button creates the claims. MediSoft will create a file of matching claims but will only include those that have not yet been billed.

Exercise 9-1

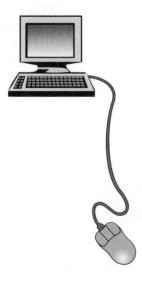

Create insurance claims for all patients who have transactions not already placed on a claim.

Date: October 5, 2004

1. Start MediSoft. Change the date if necessary.
2. On the Activities menu, click Claim Management. The Claim Management dialog box is displayed.
3. Click the Create Claims button.
4. Leave all boxes in the Create Claims dialog box blank to select all transactions.
5. Click the Create button.
6. Use the scroll bars to view the claims just created.
7. Click the Close button.

CLAIM SELECTION

At times it is necessary to select and view specific claims that have already been created. For example, any claims prepared for submission to an insurance carrier must be selected and then reviewed for completeness and accuracy. In addition, all claims that have been rejected by insurance carriers are selected and reviewed before resubmission.

MediSoft's List Only feature is used when it is necessary to list claims that match certain criteria. Filters are applied in the List Only Claims That Match dialog box. They can be used to view claims selectively, such as claims for a specific insurance carrier, claims created on a certain date, and so on. Unlike the filters in the Create Claims dialog box, those in the List Only Claims That Match dialog box do not create claims; they simply list existing claims that meet the specified criteria.

Once the filters have been applied, only those claims that match the criteria are listed at the bottom of the main Claim Management dialog box. Claims can be sorted by chart number, date the claim was created, insurance carrier, electronic media claim (EMC) receiver, billing method, billing date, batch number, and claim status. Not all the boxes need to be filled in, only the ones that will be used to select the desired claims.

The List Only feature is activated by clicking the List Only... button in the Claim Management dialog box. This causes the List Only Claims That Match dialog box to be displayed (see Figure 9-5).

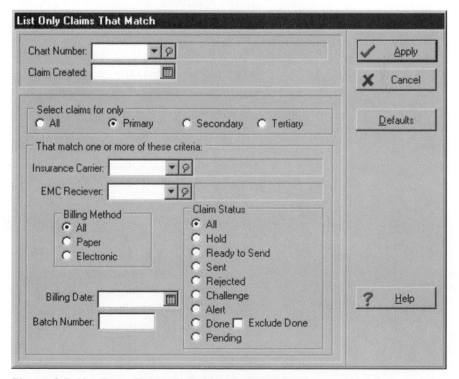

Figure 9-5 **List Only Claims That Match dialog box.**

The following filters are available in the List Only Claims That Match dialog box.

Chart Number   A patient's chart number is selected from the drop-down list of patients' chart numbers.

Claim Created   The date that a claim was created is entered in MMDDCCYY format.

Select Claims for Only   A radio button is clicked for either all insurance carriers, primary insurance carrier only, secondary insurance carrier only, or tertiary insurance carrier only. When a patient has insurance coverage with more than one carrier, the primary carrier is billed first, and then, if appropriate, the second and third (tertiary) carriers are billed.

Insurance Carrier   An insurance carrier is selected from the drop-down list of choices.

EMC Receiver   An EMC receiver is selected from the choices on the drop-down list.

Billing Method   In the Billing Method box, the radio button for All, Paper, or Electronic is clicked.

Billing Date   The date of billing is entered in the Billing Date box.

Batch Number   A batch number is entered in the Batch Number box.

Claim Status   A claim status is selected from the list of radio buttons provided. If claims that have been billed and accepted (not rejected) are to be excluded from the search, the Exclude Done box is clicked. This causes a check mark to be displayed beside the option.

When the desired boxes have been filled in, clicking the Apply button applies the selected filters to the claims data. The Claim Management dialog box is displayed listing only those claims that match the criteria selected in the List Only Claims That Match dialog box. From the Claim Management dialog box, the claims can now be edited, printed, and mailed or transmitted electronically. To restore the List Only Claims That Match dialog box to its original settings (that is, to remove the filters selected), this dialog box is reopened, the Defaults button is clicked, and then the Apply button is clicked. All of the boxes in the dialog box will become blank, and the full list of claims is displayed again in the Claim Management dialog box.

EDITING CLAIMS

MediSoft's Claim Edit feature allows claims to be reviewed and verified on screen before they are submitted to insurance carriers for payment. With careful checking, problems can be solved before claims are sent to insurance carriers. When a claim is active in the Claim Management dialog box, it can be edited by clicking the Edit button or by double-clicking the claim itself. The Claim dialog box is displayed (see Figure 9-6). The top section of the Claim dialog box lists the claim number, the date the claim was created, the chart number, the patient's name, and the case number. This information cannot be edited, although the information in the five tabs can be edited.

CARRIER 1 TAB The Carrier 1 tab displays information about claims being submitted to a patient's primary insurance carrier.

The following boxes are listed in the Carrier 1 tab:

Claim Status The Claim Status box indicates the status of a particular claim: Hold, Ready to send, Sent, Rejected, Challenge, Alert, Done, and Pending. The radio button that reflects a claim's status should be clicked.

Billing Method The Billing Method box displays two choices: Paper or Electronic. The radio button that describes the billing method should be clicked.

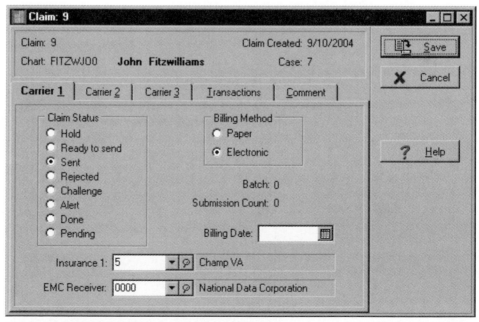

Figure 9-6 **Claim dialog box.**

Batch   If the claim has been assigned to a batch, the batch number is displayed.

Submission Count   The Submission Count area lists the number of claims submitted.

Billing Date   The Billing Date box lists the date the bill was sent.

Insurance 1   The Insurance 1 box lists a patient's primary insurance carrier.

EMC Receiver   The EMC receiver is selected from the drop-down list.

CARRIER 2 AND CARRIER 3 TABS   The Carrier 2 and Carrier 3 tabs display information about claims being submitted to a patient's secondary (Carrier 2) and tertiary (Carrier 3) insurance carriers. The boxes in these tabs are the same as the boxes in the Carrier 1 tab.

TRANSACTIONS TAB   The Transactions tab lists information about the transactions included in a claim. The scroll bars can be used to view all the information in the Transactions tab (see Figure 9-7).

Date From   The Date From box lists the date on which service was provided.

Document   The Document box lists the document number of a transaction.

Procedure   The Procedure box displays the procedure code for a procedure performed.

Amount   In the Amount box, the dollar cost of a service is displayed.

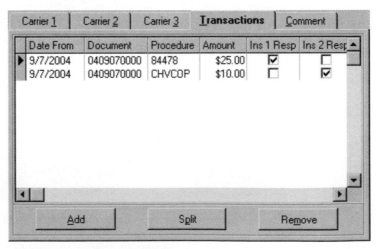

Figure 9-7 **Transactions tab.**

Ins 1 Resp If this box is checked, the primary insurance carrier is responsible for the claim.

Ins 2 Resp If this box is checked, the secondary insurance carrier is responsible for the claim.

Ins 3 Resp If this box is checked, the tertiary insurance carrier is responsible for the claim.

The Transactions tab also contains three buttons at the bottom of the dialog box: Add, Split, and Remove. The Add button is used to add a transaction to an existing claim. The Split button removes a single transaction from an existing claim and places it on a new claim. The Remove button deletes a transaction from the database.

COMMENT TAB The Comment tab provides a place to include any specific notes or comments about the claim (see Figure 9-8).

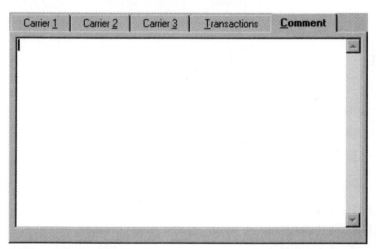

Figure 9-8 **Comment tab.**

Exercise 9-2

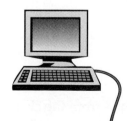

Review insurance claims for patients with East Ohio PPO as their insurance carrier.

Date: October 5, 2004

1. **Open the Claim Management dialog box.**

2. **Click the List Only... button.**

3. **Click 13 East Ohio PPO on the drop-down list in the Insurance Carrier box.**

4. **Click the Apply button. You are returned to the Claim Management dialog box. Notice that only claims for patients who have East Ohio PPO as their insurance carrier are listed.**

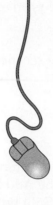

5. Double-click Chart Number BELLSAR∅ or select this chart number and click the Edit button to review the claim for Sarina Bell. The Claim dialog box is displayed.

6. Review the information in the Carrier 1 tab.

7. Review the information in the Transactions tab.

8. Click the Cancel button to exit the Claim dialog box without saving any changes. (The Cancel button does not cancel the claim; it just cancels any changes that may have been made.)

9. Close the Claim Management dialog box.

ELECTRONIC MEDIA CLAIMS

Many of the setup and entry requirements for electronic media claims (EMC) are typically handled by the medical office's systems manager. Insurance carriers and clearinghouses that receive claims electronically have different requirements regarding what information needs to be included on an electronic claim. Each insurance carrier has specific data requirements, indicating which boxes are mandatory and what the data format should be. The office systems manager maintains detailed information on the EMC requirements of each carrier and updates this information as necessary. However, some basic steps that need to be followed to submit electronic claims are common to most insurance carriers.

STEPS IN SUBMITTING ELECTRONIC CLAIMS

There are a number of steps in the process of submitting electronic claims.

1. Enter information about a patient in the usual manner.

2. Check to make sure all the information required by an insurance carrier is complete; otherwise, the claim will be rejected.

3. Enter transactions and payments as usual.

4. Create claims either through the Transaction Entry dialog box or through the Claim Management feature.

5. Review claims through the Claims Edit and the List Only features to locate any obvious errors.

6. Transmit claims to the clearinghouse.

7. Review the audit/edit report that arrives from the clearinghouse. The audit/edit report lists any problems with the claims. Correct and resubmit any claims that have errors.

8. The clearinghouse transmits the claims to an insurance carrier. The information is received by the insurance carrier and stored in its database, awaiting processing.

TRANSMITTING ELECTRONIC CLAIMS

After making sure all the information is complete and correct for claims being sent, the Print/Send button in the Claim Management dialog box is clicked. This causes the Print/Send Claims dialog box to be displayed. Within this dialog box, the billing method (paper or electronic) must be indicated (see Figure 9-9). If the claims being sent are paper, the Paper radio button is clicked. If the claims are being submitted electronically, the Electronic radio button is clicked.

When the Electronic radio button is clicked, the Electronic Claim Receiver box becomes active. The EMC receiver is selected from the list of choices in the drop-down list. After the EMC receiver has been selected and the OK button is clicked, the Send Electronic Claims dialog box is displayed (see Figure 9-10). This dialog box provides the option of sending claims now or sending claims later, via the Send Claims Now and Send Claims Later buttons. After claims are sent, the system marks them "Sent."

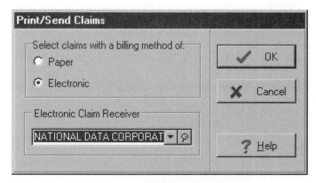

Figure 9-9 **Print/Send Claims dialog box.**

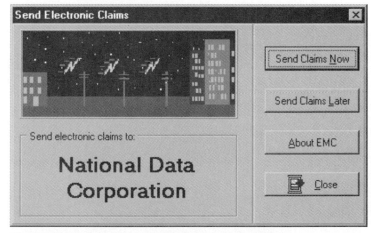

Figure 9-10 **Send Electronic Claims dialog box.**

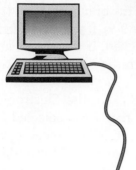

Exercise 9-3

Prepare to send electronic claims to a clearinghouse.

October 5, 2004

1. Open the Claim Management dialog box, and click the Print/Send button.

2. In the Print/Send Claims dialog box, select claims with an electronic billing method by clicking the Electronic radio button.

3. Click National Data Corporation on the drop-down list in the Electronic Claim Receiver box.

4. Click the OK button. The Send Electronic Claims dialog box is displayed.

5. If you were in a medical office and ready to send claims, you would click the Send Claims Now button. However, because you are in a school setting and are not actually set up to submit electronic claims, click the Close button.

6. Close the Claim Management dialog box.

REVIEWING THE AUDIT/EDIT REPORT

When claims are transmitted to a clearinghouse, an audit/edit report is received immediately after claims are sent (see Figure 9-11). Options for viewing and printing the report are listed on-screen when the report is received. It is important to print a copy of the report, since some systems do not permit reports to be viewed online at a later time.

The audit/edit report marks each claim as accepted or rejected. Each claim is displayed on a separate line of the report. The Message column queries whether a claim will be sent to an insurance carrier. If a claim cannot be sent, the error is listed in the Message column. In the Flag column of the report, a "P" indicates that the claim will be sent on paper; an "R" indicates that the claim was rejected. A blank Flag column means that the claim will be sent electronically. The report should be reviewed carefully. Any errors found by a clearinghouse must be corrected before a claim can be sent to an insurance carrier.

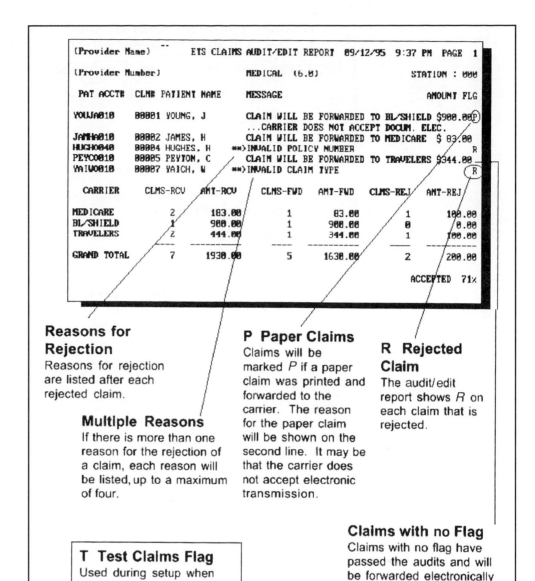

```
(Provider Name)  --        ETS CLAIMS AUDIT/EDIT REPORT  09/12/95  9:37 PM  PAGE  1

(Provider Number)               MEDICAL  (6.0)                STATION : 000

 PAT ACCT#  CLM# PATIENT NAME     MESSAGE                          AMOUNT FLG

YOUJA010  00001 YOUNG, J        CLAIM WILL BE FORWARDED TO BL/SHIELD $900.00(P)
                                ...CARRIER DOES NOT ACCEPT DOCUM. ELEC.
JAMHA010  00002 JAMES, H        CLAIM WILL BE FORWARDED TO MEDICARE  $ 83.00
HUGH0040  00004 HUGHES, H   **>INVALID POLICY NUMBER                        R
PEYCO010  00005 PEYTON, C       CLAIM WILL BE FORWARDED TO TRAVELERS $344.00
YAIVO010  00007 YAICH, W    **>INVALID CLAIM TYPE                          (R)

  CARRIER      CLMS-RCV   AMT-RCV    CLMS-FWD   AMT-FWD   CLMS-REJ   AMT-REJ

MEDICARE         2        183.00        1        83.00       1       100.00
BL/SHIELD        1        900.00        1       900.00       0         0.00
TRAVELERS        2        444.00        1       344.00       1       100.00
              -----    ----------    -----  ----------    -----   ----------
GRAND TOTAL      7       1930.00        5      1630.00       2       200.00

                                                           ACCEPTED  71%
```

Figure 9-11 **Audit/Edit report.**

Reasons for Rejection

Reasons for rejection are listed after each rejected claim.

Multiple Reasons

If there is more than one reason for the rejection of a claim, each reason will be listed, up to a maximum of four.

P Paper Claims

Claims will be marked *P* if a paper claim was printed and forwarded to the carrier. The reason for the paper claim will be shown on the second line. It may be that the carrier does not accept electronic transmission.

R Rejected Claim

The audit/edit report shows *R* on each claim that is rejected.

T Test Claims Flag

Used during setup when testing claims with a carrier. Data will not be forwarded to the carrier.

Claims with no Flag

Claims with no flag have passed the audits and will be forwarded electronically to the appropriate carrier.

Exercise 9-4

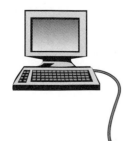

An audit/edit report has come back from the clearinghouse. A claim for James Smith has been rejected for submission to Blue Cross/Blue Shield. There are two reasons listed for rejection: "Missing Insured's ID no." and "Missing Insured's Group no." Locate the problem in MediSoft, correct it, and prepare the claim for resubmission.

Date: October 5, 2004

1. Go to the Policy 1 tab in the Case dialog box to check whether Mr. Smith's insurance policy number and group number have been entered.

2. Notice that these boxes are blank. Someone forgot to enter data in them when creating the case for Mr. Smith.

3. Key *354691* in the Policy Number box.

4. Key *U339* in the Group Number box.

5. Click the Save button.

6. Close the Patient List dialog box.

7. Open the Claim Management dialog box.

8. Double-click the rejected claim in the Claim Management dialog box to edit the claim.

9. Change the claim status from Rejected to Ready to Send. Click the Save button.

10. Close the Claim Management dialog box. (In an actual office setting, the claim would now be resent to the clearinghouse. Because schools are not set up to transmit electronic media claims, this exercise ends without actually transmitting claims.)

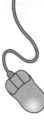

11. Exit MediSoft.

CHAPTER REVIEW

USING TERMINOLOGY

Define the terms below.

1. filter

_____

_____

2. navigator buttons

_____

_____

CHECKING YOUR UNDERSTANDING

Answer the questions below in the space provided.

3. A claim needs to be submitted for John Fitzwilliams. How would you select only those claims pertaining to John Fitzwilliams?

_____

_____

4. On an audit/edit report, what does an "R" in the Flag column indicate?

_____

_____

5. If an error is found on a claim, how is it corrected?

_____

_____

APPLYING KNOWLEDGE

Answer the question below in the space provided.

6. You were asked to create claims for Samuel Bell. After entering his chart number in the Create Claims dialog box, you receive the message "No new claims were created." Why were no claims created for Samuel Bell?

_____

_____

_____

_____

AT THE COMPUTER

Answer the following questions at the computer.

7. How many claims were created on September 10, 2004?

_____

8. What transactions were included on Jonathan Bell's claim that was created on September 10, 2004?

_____

_____

_____

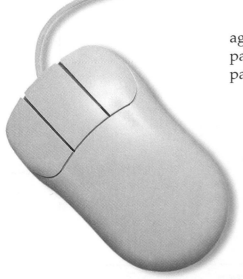

CHAPTER

10

Printing Reports

WHAT YOU NEED TO KNOW

To use this chapter, you need to know how to:
- ◆ Start MediSoft, use menus, and enter and edit text.
- ◆ Work with chart numbers and codes.

OBJECTIVES

In this chapter, you will learn how to:
- ◆ Select the options available for different reports.
- ◆ Preview and print a variety of MediSoft reports.
- ◆ Access MediSoft's Report Designer.

KEY TERMS

aging report
patient day sheet
patient ledger

patient statement
procedure day sheet

REPORTS IN THE MEDICAL OFFICE

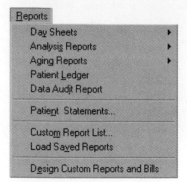

Figure 10-1 **Reports menu.**

Reports are an important tool in managing a medical office. They provide useful information about a practice and its patients. Providers and office managers ask for different reports at different times. Some providers want to see a daily report of each day's transactions. Others want to see reports on particular patients' accounts on a weekly or bimonthly basis.

MediSoft provides a variety of standard reports, and has the ability to create custom reports using the Report Designer. Standard and custom reports are accessed through the Reports menu (see Figure 10-1). The Reports menu lists standard reports and also provides choices for designing custom reports using the Report Designer.

The standard reports are day sheets, analysis reports, aging reports, patient ledger, data audit report, and patient statements.

PATIENT DAY SHEET

patient day sheet a summary of the activity of patient accounts on any given day.

At the end of the day, many medical practices print a **patient day sheet**, which is a summary of the activity of patient activity on any given day (see Figures 10-2a and 10-2b). MediSoft's version of this report lists the procedures for a particular day, grouped by patient, in alphabetical order by chart number. It includes:

Family Care Center
Patient Day Sheet
9/6/2004 - 09/06/2004

Entry	Date	Document	POS	Description	Provider	Code	Amount
ARLENSU0		**Susan Arlen**					
195	9/6/2004	0409060000			5	EAPCOPAY	-15.00
194	9/6/2004	0409060000	11		5	99212	46.00
		Patient's Charges		Patient's Receipts	Adjustments		Patient Balance
		$46.00		-$15.00	$0.00		$31.00
BELLHER0		**Herbert Bell**					
71	9/6/2004	0409060000	11		2	99211	30.00
170	9/6/2004	0409060000			2	EAPCOPAY	-15.00
		Patient's Charges		Patient's Receipts	Adjustments		Patient Balance
		$30.00		-$15.00	$0.00		$15.00
BELLJAN0		**Janine Bell**					
171	9/6/2004	0409060000			3	EAPCOPAY	-15.00
74	9/6/2004	0409060000	11		3	99213	62.00
75	9/6/2004	0409060000	11		3	73510	103.00
		Patient's Charges		Patient's Receipts	Adjustments		Patient Balance
		$165.00		-$15.00	$0.00		$150.00
BELLJON0		**Jonathan Bell**					
78	9/6/2004	0409060000	11		3	99394	149.00
172	9/6/2004	0409060000			3	EAPCOPAY	-15.00
		Patient's Charges		Patient's Receipts	Adjustments		Patient Balance
		$149.00		-$15.00	$0.00		$134.00
BELLSAM0		**Samuel Bell**					
81	9/6/2004	0409060000	11		2	99212	46.00
173	9/6/2004	0409060000			2	EAPCOPAY	-15.00
		Patient's Charges		Patient's Receipts	Adjustments		Patient Balance
		$46.00		-$15.00	$0.00		$31.00
BELLSAR0		**Sarina Bell**					
84	9/6/2004	0409060000	11		3	99213	62.00
174	9/6/2004	0409060000			3	EAPCOPAY	-15.00
		Patient's Charges		Patient's Receipts	Adjustments		Patient Balance
		$62.00		-$15.00	$0.00		$47.00

Figure 10-2a **Page 1 of Patient Day Sheet report.**

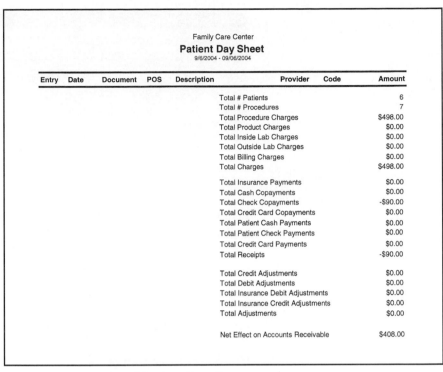

Family Care Center

Patient Day Sheet

9/6/2004 - 09/06/2004

Entry	Date	Document	POS	Description	Provider	Code	Amount
				Total # Patients			6
				Total # Procedures			7
				Total Procedure Charges			$498.00
				Total Product Charges			$0.00
				Total Inside Lab Charges			$0.00
				Total Outside Lab Charges			$0.00
				Total Billing Charges			$0.00
				Total Charges			$498.00
				Total Insurance Payments			$0.00
				Total Cash Copayments			$0.00
				Total Check Copayments			-$90.00
				Total Credit Card Copayments			$0.00
				Total Patient Cash Payments			$0.00
				Total Patient Check Payments			$0.00
				Total Credit Card Payments			$0.00
				Total Receipts			-$90.00
				Total Credit Adjustments			$0.00
				Total Debit Adjustments			$0.00
				Total Insurance Debit Adjustments			$0.00
				Total Insurance Credit Adjustments			$0.00
				Total Adjustments			$0.00
				Net Effect on Accounts Receivable			$408.00

Figure 10-2b **Page 2 of Patient Day Sheet report.**

◆ Procedures performed for a particular patient or group of patients.

◆ Charges, receipts, adjustments, and balances for a particular patient or group of patients.

◆ A summary of a practice's charges, payments, and adjustments.

To print a patient day sheet, Day Sheets is clicked on the Reports menu and Patient Day Sheet on the submenu (see Figure 10-3). Then, the Print Report Where? dialog box is displayed, asking whether the report should be previewed on the screen or sent directly to the printer (see Figure 10-4 on page 190). Reports that are previewed on the screen can also be printed from the Preview Report window.

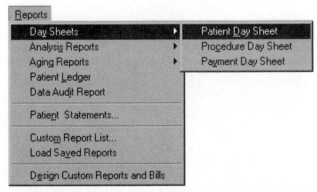

Figure 10-3 **Reports menu with Day Sheets submenu displayed.**

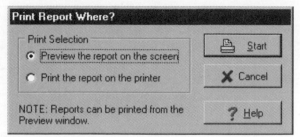

Figure 10-4 **Print Report Where? dialog box.**

When the Preview the Report on the Screen radio button is selected and the Start button is clicked, the Data Selection Questions dialog box is displayed (see Figure 10-5). This dialog box is used to select the patients, dates, and providers for whom a report is being generated. If any box is left blank, all values are included in the report. For example, if no chart numbers are entered, all patients will be included in the report. The selection options in the dialog box are as follows.

Chart Number Range   In the Chart Number Range boxes, a range of chart numbers for patients is entered. If a report is needed for just one patient, that patient's chart number is entered in both boxes.

Date Created Range   A range of dates when transactions were entered in MediSoft is entered in the two boxes. The current date is the default entry. If this is not the date desired, it can be changed by selecting new dates and entering them.

Date From Range   A range of dates is entered in the Date From Range boxes. For example, if it were necessary to print patient day sheets for the period of May 1 to May 15, 2004, "05012004" would be entered in the first box and "05152004" in the second box. If transactions were needed for the current date, that date would be entered in both boxes.

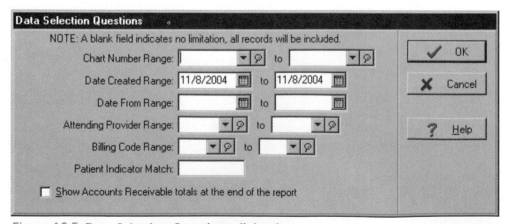

Figure 10-5 **Data Selection Questions dialog box.**

Attending Provider Range A range of codes for the attending providers is entered in the Attending Provider Range boxes.

Billing Code Range If the practice uses MediSoft's Billing Code feature, codes can be entered in this box to select only those patients with the designated billing code(s).

Patient Indicator Match If the practice has assigned a Patient Indicator code to each patient, an entry can be made to select only those patients who match a specific code.

Show Accounts Receivable Totals at the End of the Report If this box is checked, accounts receivable totals will appear at the end of the Patient Day Sheet report.

When these selection boxes have been completed, the OK button is clicked. MediSoft begins creating the report. MediSoft generates the report and displays it on-screen or sends it to the printer, depending on the selection made in the Print Report Where? dialog box.

The Preview Report window, common to all reports, provides options for viewing or printing a report (see Figure 10-6). The buttons on the

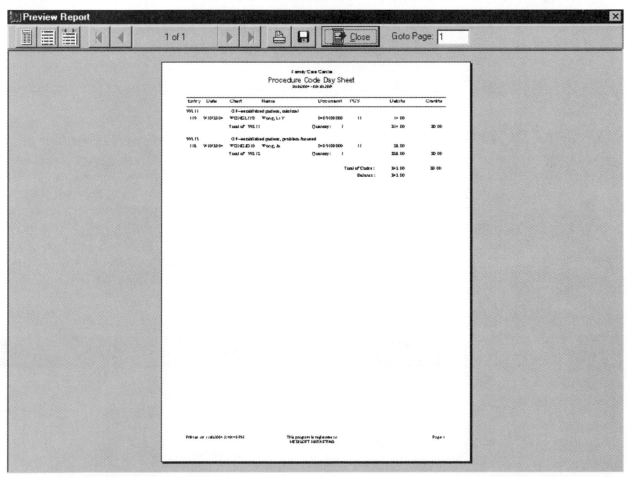

Figure 10-6 Preview Report window.

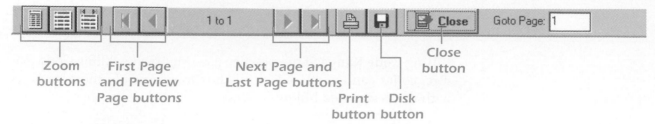

| Zoom buttons | First Page and Preview Page buttons | Next Page and Last Page buttons | Print button | Disk button | Close button |

Figure 10-7 **Buttons on Preview Report toolbar.**

Preview Report toolbar control how a report is displayed on-screen and how movement is done from page to page within a report (see Figure 10-7).

The three zoom buttons at the left of the toolbar are used to affect the size of the report displayed on-screen. The zoom button farthest to the left reduces a report so that a full page fits on the screen. The middle zoom button displays a report at 100 percent of its size. This option acts like a magnifying glass, allowing a portion of a report to be viewed up close. The zoom button on the right displays the full width of a page on the screen.

A series of four triangle buttons, two on the left and two on the right, are used to move through pages of a multipage report. The First Page button, farthest on the left, moves to the beginning of a report. The Previous Page button moves to the page that precedes the one currently displayed. The bar between the two sets of triangle buttons indicates how many pages are in a report and the number of the current page. To the right of the bar are the other two triangle buttons. The Next Page button moves to the page following the current one. The Last Page button moves to the end of a report.

The remaining buttons include the Print button, which is used to send a report to the printer, and the Disk button, which saves a report to disk. The Close button closes the Preview Report window, redisplaying the main MediSoft window.

The Preview Report window also contains the Go to Page box, in which the number of a specific page to be displayed in the Preview Report window is entered.

Exercise 10-1

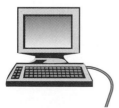

Print a patient day sheet report for July 12, 2004.

Date: July 12, 2004

1. **Start MediSoft.**

2. **On the Reports menu, click Day Sheets and then Patient Day Sheet. The Print Report Where? dialog box is displayed.**

3. Click the radio button for previewing the report on-screen if it is not already selected. Click the Start button. The Data Selection Questions dialog box is displayed.

4. Leave the Chart Number Range boxes blank. Key *07122004* in both of the Date Created Range boxes. Do not key any slashes between the numbers; MediSoft does this automatically. (Today's date—that is, the date on which you are working on this exercise, will most likely appear in both Date Created Range boxes. Select each entry and enter the July 12, 2004, date instead.) Leave all other boxes blank. This will select data for all patients and attending providers for July 12, 2004.

5. Click the OK button. The patient day sheet report is displayed.

6. Click the appropriate zoom button on the toolbar to display the report the full width of the screen so that it is easier to read.

7. Scroll down the page to view additional entries on the first page of the report.

8. Click the Next Page button to advance to the second page of the report.

9. Click the other zoom and triangle buttons on the toolbar to see their effects. Use the Go to Page box to move back to page one of the report.

10. Click the Print button, and then click the OK button on the Print menu to print the report.

11. Click the Close button to exit the Preview Report window.

PROCEDURE DAY SHEET

procedure day sheet a list of all the procedures performed on a particular day.

A **procedure day sheet** lists all of the procedures performed on a particular day, and gives the dates, patients, document numbers, places of service, debits, and credits relating to these procedures (see Figure 10-8 on page 194). Procedures are listed in numerical order. Procedure day sheets are printed by clicking Procedure Day Sheet on the Reports menu. The same Print Report Where? dialog box used for a patient day sheet is displayed. Again, the report can be previewed on-screen or printed directly.

Once the decision to preview or print is made, the data selection criteria must be determined. The Data Selection Questions dialog box provides options to select by procedure codes, dates, and providers (see Figure 10-9 on page 195). A procedure day sheet will be generated only for the data that meets the selection criteria. If any box is left blank, all values are included in the report.

Family Care Center

Procedure Code Day Sheet

9/6/2004 - 09/06/2004

Entry	Date	Chart	Name	Document	POS	Debits	Credits
73510		**hip x-ray, complete, two views**					
75	9/6/2004	BELLJAN0	Bell, Janine	0409060000	11	103.00	
		Total of 73510		Quantity: 1		$103.00	$0.00
99211		**OF--established patient, minimal**					
71	9/6/2004	BELLHER0	Bell, Herbert	0409060000	11	30.00	
		Total of 99211		Quantity: 1		$30.00	$0.00
99212		**OF--established patient, problem focused**					
81	9/6/2004	BELLSAM0	Bell, Samuel	0409060000	11	46.00	
194	9/6/2004	ARLENSU0	Arlen, Susan	0409060000	11	46.00	
		Total of 99212		Quantity: 2		$92.00	$0.00
99213		**OF--established patient, expanded**					
84	9/6/2004	BELLSAR0	Bell, Sarina	0409060000	11	62.00	
74	9/6/2004	BELLJAN0	Bell, Janine	0409060000	11	62.00	
		Total of 99213		Quantity: 2		$124.00	$0.00
99394		**established patient, adolescent, per...**					
78	9/6/2004	BELLJON0	Bell, Jonathan	0409060000	11	149.00	
		Total of 99394		Quantity: 1		$149.00	$0.00
EAPCOPAY		**East Ohio PPO Copayment**					
171	9/6/2004	BELLJAN0	Bell, Janine	0409060000			-15.00
170	9/6/2004	BELLHER0	Bell, Herbert	0409060000			-15.00
172	9/6/2004	BELLJON0	Bell, Jonathan	0409060000			-15.00
173	9/6/2004	BELLSAM0	Bell, Samuel	0409060000			-15.00
174	9/6/2004	BELLSAR0	Bell, Sarina	0409060000			-15.00
195	9/6/2004	ARLENSU0	Arlen, Susan	0409060000			-15.00
		Total of EAPCOPAY		Quantity: 6		$0.00	-$90.00
					Total of Codes:	$498.00	-$90.00
					Balance:	$408.00	

Figure 10-8 **Procedure Day Sheet report.**

The following boxes are listed in the Data Selection Questions dialog box.

Procedure Code Range In the Procedure Code Range box, a range of procedure codes is entered. If a report is needed for a single code, it is entered in both boxes.

Date Created Range A range of dates when transactions were entered in MediSoft is entered in the two boxes. The Windows system date is the default entry. If this is not the date desired, it can be changed by selecting new dates and entering them.

Date From Range A range of dates when each transaction occurred is entered in the Date From Range boxes.

Attending Provider Range Codes for attending providers are entered in the Attending Provider Range boxes.

Show Accounts Receivable Totals at the End of the Report If this box is checked, accounts receivable totals will appear at the end of the report.

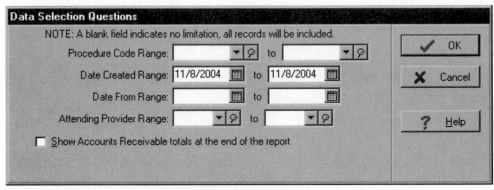

Figure 10-9 **Data Selection Questions dialog box.**

Exercise 10-2

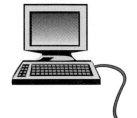

Print a procedure day sheet report for July 12, 2004, with the entire range of procedure codes, dates from, and attending providers.

Date: July 12, 2004

1. **On the Reports menu, click Day Sheets and then Procedure Day Sheet. The Print Report Where? dialog box is displayed.**

2. **Click the radio button option for previewing the report on-screen. Click the Start button. The Data Selection Questions dialog box is displayed.**

3. **Leave the Procedure Code Range boxes blank.**

4. **Key** *07122004* **in both Date Created Range boxes. Leave the other boxes blank. Click the OK button. The procedure day sheet report is displayed.**

5. **Send the report to the printer.**

6. **Exit the Preview Report window.**

PRACTICE MediSoft's practice analysis report analyzes the revenue of a prac-
ANALYSIS tice for a specified period of time, usually a month or a year (see
REPORT Figures 10-10a and 10-10b on page 196). The report can be used to
generate medical practice financial statements. It can also be used
for profit analysis. The summary at the end of the report breaks
down the report into total charges, total lab charges (both inside and
outside), total patient payments, copayments, credit card payments,
insurance payments, and total credits and debits by both patient and
insurance. The following boxes are listed in the Data Selection
Questions dialog box (see Figure 10-11 on page 196).

Family Care Center
Practice Analysis
From September 1, 2004 to September 30, 2004

Code	Description	Amount	Quantity	Average	Cost	Net
29425	application of short leg cast, walking	75.00	1	75.00	0.00	75.00
50390	aspiration of renal cyst by needle	133.00	1	133.00	0.00	133.00
73510	hip x-ray, complete, two views	103.00	1	103.00	0.00	103.00
84478	triglycerides test	25.00	1	25.00	0.00	25.00
90703	tetanus injection	20.00	1	20.00	0.00	20.00
92516	facial nerve function studies	142.00	1	142.00	0.00	142.00
96900	ultraviolet light treatment	15.00	1	15.00	0.00	15.00
99070	supplies and materials provided	20.00	1	20.00	0.00	20.00
99201	OF--new patient, problem focused	64.00	2	32.00	0.00	64.00
99211	OF--established patient, minimal	62.00	3	20.67	0.00	62.00
99212	OF--established patient, problem foc	278.00	7	39.71	0.00	278.00
99213	OF--established patient, expanded	124.00	2	62.00	0.00	124.00
99394	established patient, adolescent, per..	149.00	1	149.00	0.00	149.00
CHVCOP	ChampVA Copayment Charge	20.00	2	10.00	0.00	20.00
CHVCOPAY	ChampVA Copayment	-20.00	2	-10.00	0.00	-20.00
EAPCOP	East Ohio PPO Copayment Charge	120.00	8	15.00	0.00	120.00
EAPCOPAY	East Ohio PPO Copayment	-120.00	8	-15.00	0.00	-120.00
MCDCOP	Medicaid Copayment Charge	5.00	1	5.00	0.00	5.00
MCDCOPAY	Medicaid Copayment	-5.00	1	-5.00	0.00	-5.00
OHCCOP2	OhioCare HMO Copayment Charge	30.00	2	15.00	0.00	30.00
OHCCOPAY	OhioCare HMO Copayment	-30.00	2	-15.00	0.00	-30.00
TRICOP	Tricare Copayment Charge	15.00	1	15.00	0.00	15.00
TRICOPAY	Tricare Copayment	-15.00	1	-15.00	0.00	-15.00

Figure 10-10a Page 1 of Practice Analysis report.

Family Care Center
Practice Analysis
From September 1, 2004 to September 30, 2004

Code	Description	Amount	Quantity	Average	Cost	Net
			Total Procedure Charges			$1,400.00
			Total Product Charges			$0.00
			Total Inside Lab Charges			$0.00
			Total Outside Lab Charges			$0.00
			Total Billing Charges			$0.00
			Total Insurance Payments			$0.00
			Total Cash Copayments			$0.00
			Total Check Copayments			-$190.00
			Total Credit Card Copayments			$0.00
			Total Patient Cash Payments			$0.00
			Total Patient Check Payments			$0.00
			Total Credit Card Payments			$0.00
			Total Debit Adjustments			$0.00
			Total Credit Adjustments			$0.00
			Total Insurance Debit Adjustments			$0.00
			Total Insurance Credit Adjustments			$0.00
			Net Effect on Accounts Receivable			$1,210.00

Figure 10-10b Page 2 of Practice Analysis report.

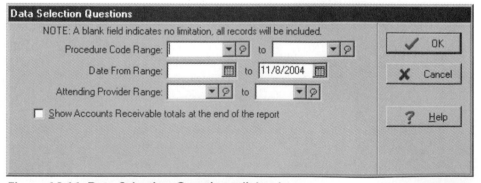

Figure 10-11 Data Selection Questions dialog box.

Procedure Code Range   A range of procedure codes is entered in the Procedure Code Range boxes.

Date From Range   A range of dates is entered in the Date From Range boxes. The system enters a default entry in the second of the two boxes. To change this date, highlight the default entry and enter the new date in MMDDCCYY format.

Attending Provider Range   Codes for attending providers are entered in the Attending Provider Range boxes.

Show Accounts Receivable Totals at the End of the Report   If this box is checked, accounts receivable totals will appear at the end of the report.

Exercise 10-3

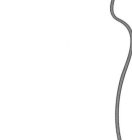

Print a practice analysis report for July 2004.

Date: July 31, 2004

1. **On the Reports menu, click Analysis Reports and then Practice Analysis.**

2. **Click the radio button for previewing the report on-screen. Click the Start button.**

3. **Leave the Procedure Code Range boxes blank.**

4. **In the first Date From Range box, key** *07012004.* **In the second box, key** *07312004.*

5. **Leave the Attending Provider Range boxes blank. Click the OK button.**

6. **View the report on-screen.**

7. **Go to the second page of the report.**

8. **Send the report to the printer.**

9. **Exit the Preview Report window.**

PATIENT AGING REPORT

aging report a report that lists the amounts owed to the practice, categorized by the number of days late.

An **aging report** lists the amount of money owed to the practice, organized by the amount of time the money has been owed. A patient aging report lists a patient's balance by age, the date of the last payment, and the telephone number. The columns display the amounts that are current and those that are 31–60, 61–90, and more than 90 days past due (see Figure 10-12 on page 198). The aging begins on the date of the transaction. Patient aging reports are printed by clicking Aging Reports and then Patient Aging on the Reports

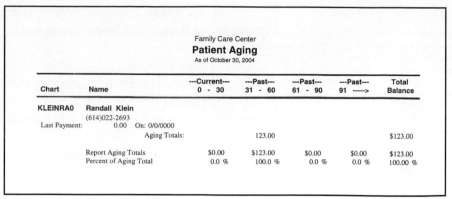

Family Care Center
Patient Aging
As of October 30, 2004

Chart	Name	---Current--- 0 - 30	---Past--- 31 - 60	---Past--- 61 - 90	---Past--- 91 ---->	Total Balance
KLEINRA0	Randall Klein					
	(614)022-2693					
Last Payment:	0.00 On: 0/0/0000					
	Aging Totals:		123.00			$123.00
	Report Aging Totals	$0.00	$123.00	$0.00	$0.00	$123.00
	Percent of Aging Total	0.0 %	100.0 %	0.0 %	0.0 %	100.00 %

Figure 10-12 **Patient Aging report.**

menu. After making a selection in the Print Report Where? dialog box, the data must be selected. The boxes in the Data Selection Questions dialog box are as follows (See Figure 10-13).

Chart Number Range   In the Chart Number Range boxes, a range of chart numbers for patients is entered. If the report is needed for just one patient, that patient's chart number is entered in both boxes.

Date From Range   A range of dates is entered in the Date From Range boxes. The system enters a default entry in the second of the two boxes. To change this date, highlight the default entry and enter the new date in MMDDCCYY format.

Attending Provider Range   A range of codes for the attending providers is entered in the Attending Provider Range boxes.

Billing Code Range If the practice uses MediSoft's Billing Code feature, codes can be entered in this box to select only those patients with the designated billing code(s).

Patient Indicator Match   If the practice has assigned a Patient Indicator code to each patient, an entry can be made to select only those patients who match a specific code.

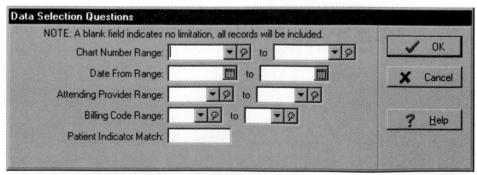

Figure 10-13 **Data Selection Questions dialog box.**

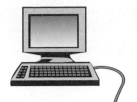

Exercise 10-4

Print a patient aging report for Jo Wong.

Date: September 30, 2004

1. On the Reports menu, click Aging Reports and then Patient Aging.

2. Click the radio button for previewing the report on-screen. Click the Start button.

3. Select Wong's chart number in both boxes of the Chart Number Range boxes.

4. Leave the starting date in the first of the Date From Range boxes blank, and key *09302004* in the second of the boxes.

5. Leave the Attending Provider Range boxes blank. Click the OK button.

6. View the report on-screen.

7. Print the report.

8. Exit the Preview Report window.

INSURANCE AGING REPORT

An insurance aging report permits tracking of claims filed with insurance carriers. The report lists claims that have been on file 0–30 days, 31–60 days, 61–90 days, and 91–999 days (see Figure 10-14 on page 200). This information is used to follow up on overdue payments from insurance carriers. Printing the aging report and following up on overdue claims speeds the collection process. The aging begins on the date of billing. MediSoft provides three insurance aging reports: primary, secondary, and tertiary. Boxes in the Data Selection Questions dialog box for all three reports are as follows (see Figure 10-15 on page 200).

Insurance Carrier 1 Range A range of codes for insurance carriers is entered in the Insurance Carrier 1 Range boxes.

Primary Billing Date Range A range of billing dates for the primary insurance carrier is entered in the Primary Billing Date Range boxes. The program displays the Windows System Date as the default entry in the second of these boxes.

Attending Provider Range Codes for attending providers are entered in the Attending Provider Range boxes.

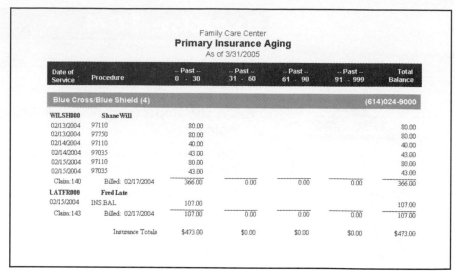

Figure 10-14 **Primary Insurance Aging report.**

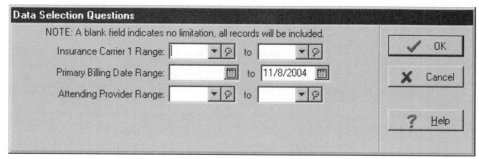

Figure 10-15 **Data Selection Questions dialog box.**

A **patient ledger** lists the financial activity in each patient's account, including charges, payments, and adjustments (see Figure 10-16). This information is especially useful if there is a question about a patient's account. A full set of patient ledgers details the status of every patient's account.

Patient ledgers are printed by clicking Patient Ledger on the Reports menu. The Print Report Where? dialog box is displayed. After the preview or print selection is made, the Data Selection Questions dialog box is displayed as it is with the other reports (see Figure 10-17). It provides options to select by chart numbers, patient reference balances, dates, and providers. A patient ledger is generated only for data that meet the selection criteria. If any selection box is left blank, all values are included in the report.

Chart Number Range   In the Chart Number Range box, a range of chart numbers for patients is entered. If a report is needed for just one patient, that patient's chart number is entered in both boxes.

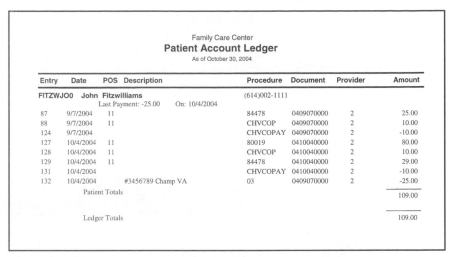

Figure 10-16 **Patient Account Ledger report.**

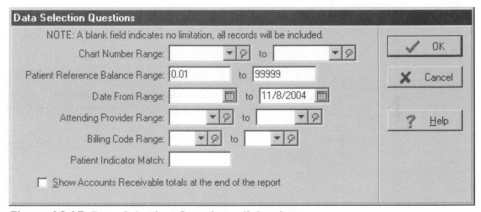

Figure 10-17 **Data Selection Questions dialog box.**

Patient Reference Balance Range   Minimum and maximum dollar amounts are entered in the Patient Reference Balance Range boxes to delineate the dollar amount of an outstanding balance. The amounts are entered with decimal points.

Date From Range   A range of dates is entered in the Date From Range boxes. For example, if it were necessary to print patient day sheets for the period of May 1 to May 15, 2004, "05012004" would be entered in the first box and "05152004" in the second box. If transactions were needed for the current date, that date would be entered in both boxes.

Attending Provider Range   A range of codes for the attending providers is entered in the Attending Provider Range boxes.

Billing Code Range If the practice uses MediSoft's Billing Code feature, codes can be entered in this box to select only those patients with the designated billing code(s).

Patient Indicator Match If the practice has assigned a Patient Indicator code to each patient, an entry can be made to select only those patients who match a specific code.

Show Accounts Receivable Totals at the End of the Report If this box is checked, accounts receivable totals will appear at the end of the report.

Exercise 10-5

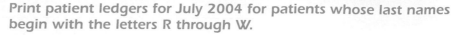

Print patient ledgers for July 2004 for patients whose last names begin with the letters R through W.

Date: July 31, 2004

1. On the Reports menu, click Patient Ledger.

2. If necessary, click the radio button for previewing the report on-screen. Click the Start button.

3. Key *R* in the first box of the Chart Number Range box and press Tab. Key *W* in the second box. Notice that the program stopped at the first patient with a last name beginning with "W." To include all patients with last names beginning with "W," key *WONGL* to select Li Wong, the last patient, and press Tab.

4. Press Tab twice to keep the default settings in the Patient Reference Balance Range boxes.

5. In the first Date From Range box, enter July 1, 2004. In the second box, enter July 31, 2004.

6. Leave the Attending Provider Range boxes blank.

7. Click the OK button.

8. Send the report to the printer.

9. Exit the Preview Report window.

PATIENT STATEMENTS

patient statement a listing of the amount of money a patient owes.

A **patient statement** lists the amount of money a patient owes, organized by the amount of time the money has been owed, the procedures performed, and the dates the procedures were performed. The bottom of the report lists total payments, total charges, total adjustments, and the balance due (see Figure 10-18). Patient statements are printed and sent out on a regular basis to patients who have an outstanding balance. Statements are not printed for patients with a zero balance on their account.

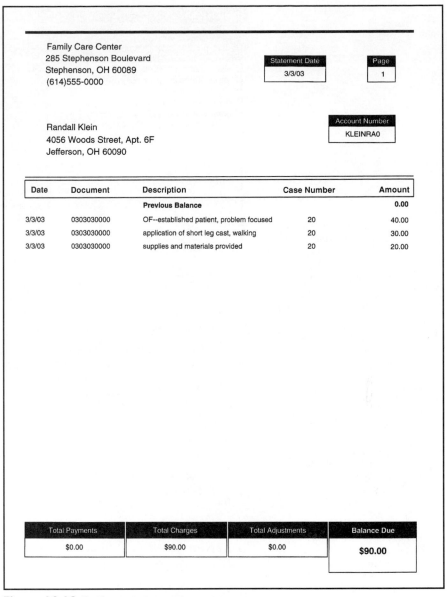

Figure 10-18 **Patient statement.**

When Patient Statements is clicked on the Reports menu, the Open Report dialog box appears (see Figure 10-19 on page 204). There are several options in the Open Report dialog box.

◆ Patient Statement (30, 60, 90).

◆ Patient Statement (Color).

◆ Patient Statement (Color) (30, 60, 90).

◆ Patient Statement.

◆ Pre-Printed Statement.

◆ Remainder Statement (All Payments).

◆ Remainder Statement (Combined Payments).

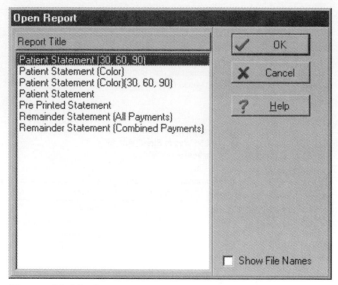

Figure 10-19 **Open Report dialog box.**

The Patient Statement (30, 60, 90) option prints the standard MediSoft patient statement. The Patient Statement (Color) option prints a color version of the standard MediSoft patient statement, assuming a color printer is used. The Pre-Printed Statement option is chosen when a medical practice uses its own preprinted forms to print patient statements. The Remainder Statements are used to print patient statements after all insurance carrier payments have been received. Like any of the standard reports in MediSoft, patient statements can be customized using MediSoft's Report Designer, discussed later in this chapter.

After the statement type is selected, the OK button is clicked. The Print Report Where? dialog box is displayed. After the choice to preview or print is made, the Data Selection Questions dialog box is displayed (see Figure 10-20). The following selections can be made.

Chart Number Range In the Chart Number Range boxes, a range of chart numbers for patients is entered. If a report is needed for just one patient, that patient's chart number is entered in both boxes.

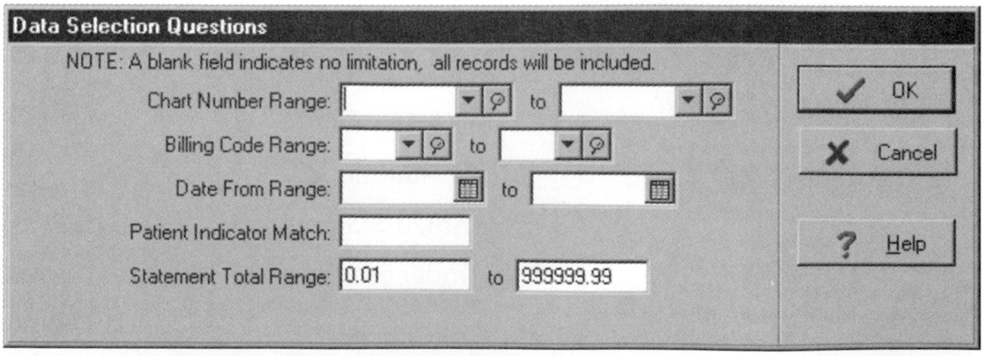

Figure 10-20 **Data Selection Questions dialog box.**

Billing Code Range A range of billing codes to be included is entered in the Billing Code Range boxes.

Date From Range A range of dates is entered in the Date From Range boxes.

Patient Indicator Match If indicator codes are used by a practice, a range of codes can be entered to select only those patients who match the indicator criteria. For example, if an indicator code has been set up to track patients receiving treatment for a certain condition, it could be entered here to limit statements printed to those patients.

Statement Total Range The Statement Total Range boxes are used to filter claims that are below a certain dollar amount. For example, the practice might have a policy of not billing patients whose account balance is less than $1.00.

Exercise 10-6

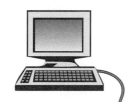

Print patient statements for July 2004 for patients whose last names begin with the letters R through W.

Date: July 31, 2004

1. On the Reports menu, click Patient Statements.

2. In the Open Report dialog box, click Patient Statement (30, 60, 90) if it is not already selected. Then click the OK button.

3. Click the radio button for previewing the report on-screen. Click the Start button.

4. Key *R* in the first Chart Number Range box and *WONGL* in the second box.

5. Leave the Billing Code Range boxes blank.

6. Enter July 1, 2004, to July 31, 2004, in the Date From Range boxes.

7. Leave all other boxes blank. Click the OK button.

8. View the report at the full width of the screen. Notice that only one statement appears. This is because the other patients who appeared on the Patient Ledger report in Exercise 10-5 have zero balances—the amount of payments is equal to the amount of the charges.

9. Send the report to the printer.

10. Exit the Preview Report window.

CUSTOM REPORTS

MediSoft has already created a number of custom reports using the built-in Report Designer. These reports include:

◆ Lists of addresses, billing codes, EMC receivers, patients, patient recalls, procedure codes, providers, and referring providers.

◆ The HCFA 1500 and the Medicare HCFA form in a variety of printer formats.

◆ Patient statements and walkout receipts.

◆ Superbills.

When Custom Report List is clicked on the Reports menu, the Open Report dialog box is displayed, listing a variety of custom reports already created in MediSoft using the Report Designer (see Figure 10-21). Additional custom reports can be created using the Report Designer. When a new custom report is created, it is added to the list of custom reports that is displayed on-screen.

The Open Report dialog box also contains six radio buttons that are used to control the list of reports displayed in the dialog box. When the All radio button is clicked, all types of custom reports are listed in the dialog box. However, when one of the other radio buttons is clicked, only reports of that style are listed. For example, if the Insurance Form radio button is clicked, only those reports that are insurance forms are listed.

To print a custom report, the title of the report is highlighted by clicking it and then the OK button is clicked. The same option that is available with standard reports for previewing the report on-screen or sending it directly to the printer is available with custom reports.

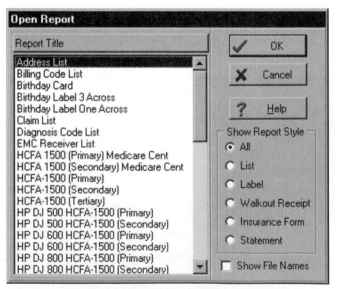

Figure 10-21 **Open Report dialog box.**

SHORT CUT To print a custom report, double-click the report title.

Exercise 10-7

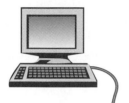

Print a list of all patients.

Date: July 31, 2004

1. On the Reports menu, click Custom Report List.

2. Select Patient List. Click the OK button.

3. Click the radio button to preview the report on-screen. Click the Start button.

4. Leave the Chart Number Range boxes blank to select all patients.

5. Click the OK button.

6. View the report on-screen.

7. Send the report to the printer.

8. Exit the Preview Report window.

Exercise 10-8

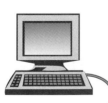

Print a list of procedure and diagnosis codes in the database.

Date: July 31, 2004

1. On the Reports menu, click Custom Report List.

2. In the Show Report Style section of the dialog box, click the List radio button.

3. Select Procedure Code List. Click the OK button.

4. Click the radio button to preview the report on-screen. Click the Start button.

5. View the report on-screen.

6. Send the report to the printer.

7. Following the same steps, print a Diagnosis Code list.

8. Exit the Preview Report window.

USING REPORT DESIGNER

Using MediSoft's Report Designer allows the user maximum flexibility and control over data in the report and how they are displayed. Formatting styles include list, ledger, statement, and insurance. Reports can be created from scratch, or an existing report can be used as a starting point. The details of how to create new custom reports with the Report Designer is beyond the coverage of this book, but Exercise 10-9 offers practice working with the Report Designer to modify an existing report. The Report Designer is accessed by clicking Design Custom Reports and Bills on the Reports menu. This action causes the Report Designer window to be displayed (see Figure 10-22).

Figure 10-22 **MediSoft's Report Designer window.**

Exercise 10-9

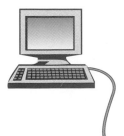

Modify the Patient List report so that a work telephone number replaces a home telephone number in the report.

Date: July 31, 2004

1. On the Reports menu, click Design Custom Reports and Bills. The Report Designer window is displayed.

2. Click Open Report on the File menu. The Open Report dialog box is displayed.

3. Double-click Patient List in the list. The Patient List report is displayed (see Figure 10-23).

4. Notice the black band that runs across the width of the window. That band contains column labels. Double-click Phone in the black bar to edit the label to read Work Phone. The Text Properties dialog box is displayed (see Figure 10-24).

5. Key *Work Phone* in the Text box that currently reads Phone.

6. Since Work Phone contains more letters than Phone, it is necessary to lengthen the space allotted for the label on the report so all the letters can be displayed. This is done in the section of the dialog box labeled Size. Click in the Auto Size box to deselect that option. In the Width box, key *120* to replace the current entry.

7. Click the OK button. Work Phone is displayed on the black band where Phone used to be.

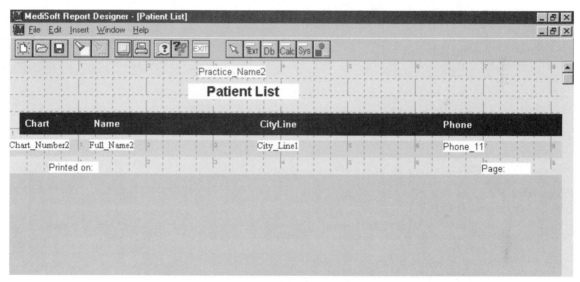

Figure 10-23 Patient List report in the MediSoft Report Designer.

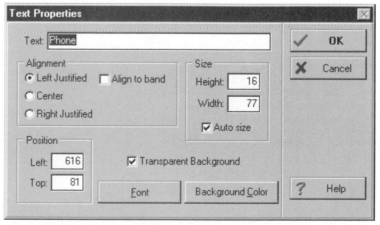

Figure 10-24 Text Properties dialog box.

8. In the green band below the black band, click the Phone 11 box to select it. Then double-click the Phone 11 box to edit its contents. The Data Field Properties dialog box is displayed (see Figure 10-25).

9. The current data box, Print Patient Phone 1, is active in the Data Field and Expressions box. Click the Edit button to change this box. The Select Data Field dialog box is displayed (see Figure 10-26).

10. In the Fields column, highlight Work Phone and click OK. The Data Field and Expressions box now lists Print Patient Work Phone.

11. To increase the space allotted in the report for this new value, click the Auto size box to deselect it. Then go to the Width box and key *120*. Click the OK button. Work Phone 1 is displayed where Phone 11 used to be.

12. On the Report Designer File menu, click Preview Report to see how the report will look when printed. The Save Report As... dialog box is displayed.

13. Key *Patient List - Work* in the Report Title box. Click the OK button. The Data Selection Questions dialog box is displayed.

14. Leave the Chart Number Range boxes blank to select all patients for the report.

15. Click the OK button.

16. The Preview Report dialog box is displayed, showing the report.

17. Click the Print button to print the report.

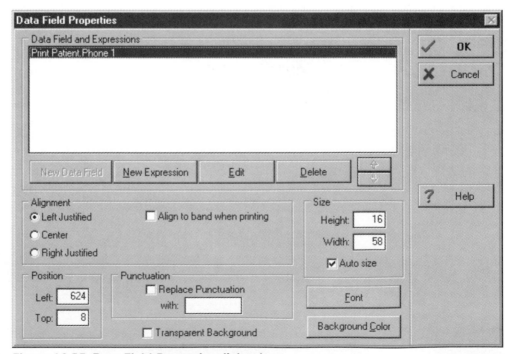

Figure 10-25 **Data Field Properties dialog box.**

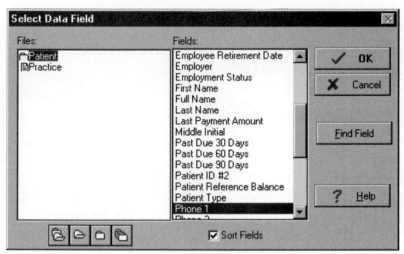

Figure 10-26 **Select Data Field dialog box.**

18. **Exit the Preview Report window.**

19. **Click Close on the Report Designer File menu, or click the Close button in the top right corner of the dialog box, to close the report file.**

20. **Click Exit on the File menu, or click the Exit button on the toolbar, to leave MediSoft's Report Designer.**

21. **Exit MediSoft.**

CHAPTER REVIEW

USING TERMINOLOGY

Match the terms on the left with the definitions on the right.

_____ **1.** aging report

_____ **2.** patient day sheet

_____ **3.** patient ledger

_____ **4.** patient statement

_____ **5.** procedure day sheet

a. A summary of the activity of a patient on any given day.

b. A report that lists procedures performed on a particular day and the dates, patients, document numbers, places of service, debits, and credits relating to these procedures.

c. A report that lists the amount of money owed, organized by the amount of time the money has been owed.

d. A report that lists the financial activity in each patient's account, including charges, payments, and adjustments.

e. A printed document that informs the patient of the amount of money owed.

CHECKING YOUR UNDERSTANDING

Answer the questions below in the space provided.

6. Which report can show the status of each patient's account on a separate page?

_____

_____

7. What is the name of the dialog box that has an option for including data on only those patients who fall within a certain chart number range?

_____

_____

8. Which report indicates how far past due a patient's account is?

_____

_____

9. Which entries print in a report if the boxes in the Data Selection Questions dialog box are left blank?

_____

_____

APPLYING KNOWLEDGE

Answer the questions below in the space provided.

10. One of the providers in a practice asks for a report of yesterday's transactions. How would this report be created?

_____

_____

11. A patient is unsure of whether or not she mailed a check last month for an outstanding balance on her account. How could you use MediSoft's Reports feature to help answer her question?

_____

_____

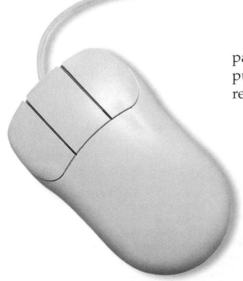

CHAPTER

11

Using Utilities

WHAT YOU NEED TO KNOW

To use this chapter, you need to know how to:
◆ Start MediSoft and use menus.
◆ Enter and edit text.

OBJECTIVES

In this chapter, you will learn how to:
◆ Make backup copies of data.
◆ View and restore backed up data.
◆ Use MediSoft's file maintenance features.

KEY TERMS

packing data   removable media device
purging data   restoring data
rebuilding indexes

MEDISOFT'S UTILITY FEATURES

MediSoft provides a number of built-in utilities to manage and maintain the data stored in the system. The utilities in MediSoft are used for saving and storing data, retrieving data, maintaining data files, and deleting data that are no longer needed. All MediSoft's utilities are accessed through the File menu.

Whenever information is stored on a computer, it is possible to lose data. The cause can be a machine failure, sometimes called a hard disk crash, or the cause can be human error, such as when data are erased accidentally by pressing the wrong key. MediSoft's backup utility can minimize the amount of data that has to be reentered should a loss of data occur. If copies of computer data files, called backups (see Chapter 3), are created on a regular basis, the amount of actual data gone from a system when a data loss occurs is minimal. It is limited to the amount entered between the time of the loss and the time the last backup was performed.

> **Warning!** Do not attempt to perform the utility functions listed in this chapter on your computer. They are for reference only. MediSoft's utility features are intended for use in a system in which data are stored on an internal hard disk. The data in this book are being stored on the Student Data Disk, a floppy disk. If the utility functions were performed, data on the Student Data Disk would be erased.

BACKING UP DATA

removable media device *a device that stores data but is not a permanent part of a computer.*

Medical offices generally have a regular schedule for backing up data. Depending on the volume of information, backups may be done as often as once a day or as infrequently as once a week. When data are backed up, they are stored on a **removable media device**. A removable media device is one that stores data but is not a permanent part of a computer. Examples of removable media devices include disks, cartridges, tapes, and CD-ROMs. Removable media devices may be stored at a location other than the office to protect them from fire or theft.

To perform a data backup in an office situation, you would complete the following steps.

1. Click Backup Data on the File menu. The MediSoft Backup dialog box is displayed (see Figure 11-1).

2. Insert the removable media device in the drive.

3. Click the Destination Path radio button that corresponds to the drive that contains the removable media device.

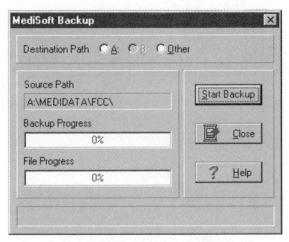

Figure 11-1 **MediSoft Backup dialog box.**

4. Click the Start Backup button. The backup proceeds automatically. When the backup is complete, the MediSoft Backup dialog box disappears from the screen and a "Backup complete" message is displayed. (To abort the backup process, the Close button is clicked.)

5. Eject the removable media device, and label it with the date and time of the backup and with any other information required by the medical office.

Viewing Backup Data

MediSoft provides a feature that allows a list of files on a backup device to be viewed on-screen or in a printed format. Information about the backup files is listed in the Backup View dialog box. In the top section of the dialog box, the following information is displayed: the name of the backup file and its location, the time and date it was created, the original data path, and the total number of files. The middle of the dialog box contains information about each file in the backup. File names, dates, times, original and compressed sizes, and the percentage of disk space saved by compression are listed.

To view backup data in an office situation, you would complete the following steps.

1. Click View Backup Disks on the File menu. The View Backup dialog box is displayed.

2. In the Source Path box, click the radio button for the drive that contains the disk or the device with the backup files.

3. Click the View Backup button. The Backup View dialog box is displayed (see Figure 11-2 on page 218).

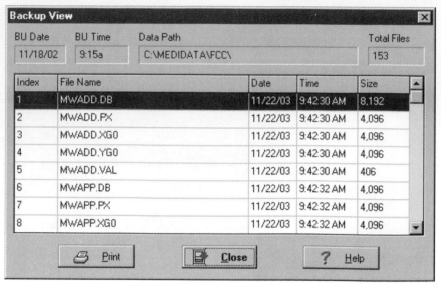

Figure 11-2 **Backup View dialog box.**

4. Review the information on-screen, or print it by clicking the Print button.

5. Click the Close button to exit the Backup View dialog box.

RESTORING DATA

restoring data *the process of retrieving data from backup storage devices.*

The process of retrieving data from backup storage devices is called **restoring data**. Data are not restored very often; only when there are serious problems with the current data is it necessary to use MediSoft's restore feature. Restoring data replaces all other data in the database. Since backup data are typically at least one day old, all the transactions, patient data, and appointments that were entered since the backup was made need to be reentered. This is one reason why it is important to print daily reports of activity in the practice. These reports can be used to reenter data when data need to be restored.

To restore data in an office situation, you would complete the following steps.

1. Click Restore Data on the File menu. A Warning box is displayed, stating that the current files are about to be overwritten. The button options in this box are OK and Cancel. If the OK button is clicked, the Restore dialog box is displayed (see Figure 11-3).

2. Insert the removable media device that contains the backup data in the drive.

3. Click the Source Path radio button that corresponds to the drive that contains the removable media device.

4. Click the Start Restore button. (To abort the Restore process, click the Close button.)

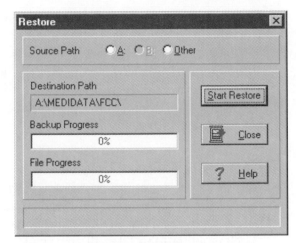

Figure 11-3 **Restore dialog box.**

5. The restore proceeds automatically. When the process is complete, the Restore dialog box disappears from the screen.

FILE MAINTENANCE UTILITIES

MediSoft provides four features to assist in maintaining data files stored in a system. These four features are found on tabs in the File Maintenance dialog box (see Figure 11-4).

◆ Rebuild Indexes.

◆ Pack Data.

◆ Purge Data.

◆ Recalculate Balances.

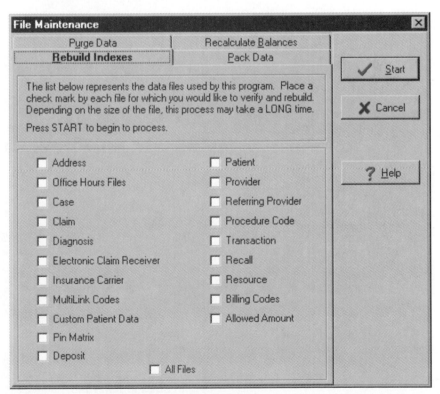

Figure 11-4 **File Maintenance dialog box.**

The dialog box is accessed by clicking File Maintenance on the File menu.

If the medical office's database is large, MediSoft's utilities may take a long time to finish. For this reason, it is usually a good idea to use the utility functions at the end of the day or when the system will not be needed for a while.

Rebuilding Indexes

rebuilding indexes a process that checks and verifies data and corrects any internal problems with the data.

Rebuilding indexes is a process that checks and verifies data and corrects any internal problems with the data. The rebuild does not check or verify the content of the data. For example, the system will not check whether John Fitzwilliams paid $50 on his last visit. Rebuilding does not change the content of any data files. To keep files working efficiently, files should be rebuilt about once a month. Files to be rebuilt are selected from the list of files in the Rebuild Indexes tab (see Figure 11-5). If the database is large, rebuilding indexes could take a long time.

To rebuild files in Medisoft in an office, you would complete the following steps.

1. Click File Maintenance on the File menu. The File Maintenance dialog box is displayed with the Rebuild Indexes tab active.
2. Click in each check box next to the files that are to be verified and rebuilt. If all files are to be rebuilt, click the All Files box at the

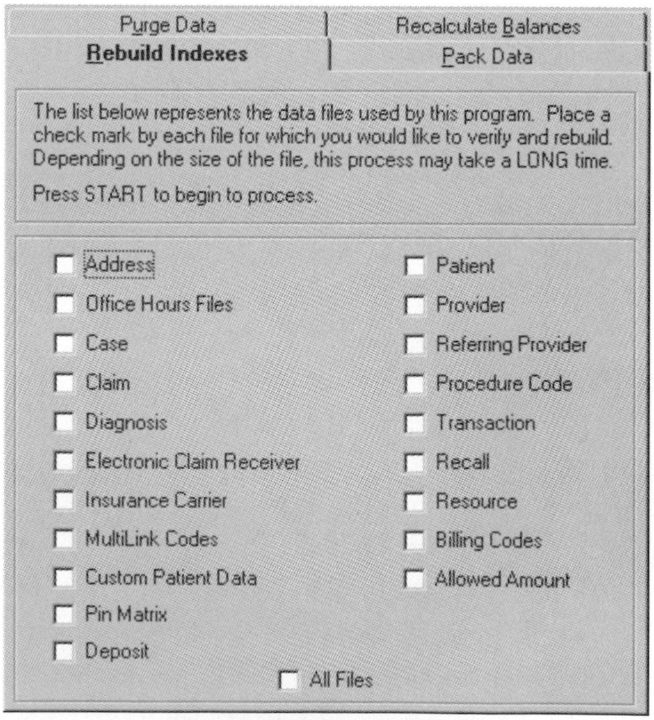

Figure 11-5 **Rebuild Indexes tab.**

bottom of the list of files. This saves the time it would take to click a box for every MediSoft file.

3. Click the Start button. The Confirm dialog box is displayed with the message "All of the checked file processes will be performed. Do you want to continue?" Click the OK button to continue. (Clicking the Cancel button aborts the process.)

4. The rebuild process is performed automatically. When the process is complete, the message "All checked file processes are complete" is displayed.

Packing Data

When data are deleted in MediSoft, the system empties the data from the record but keeps the empty slot in the database so it is available when new data need to be entered in the system. For example, if a patient were deleted in the Patient List dialog box, the system would delete all the records pertaining to that patient but would maintain an empty slot in the patient database. Then, the next time a new patient is entered, the data for the new patient would occupy the vacant slot in the database. In cases in which there is not much space available on the hard disk, it is sometimes desirable to delete the vacant slots to make more disk space available. The deletion of vacant slots from the database is known as **packing data**. Data for packing can be selected from the list of files in the Pack Data tab (see Figure 11-6). (Only transaction files with a zero balance can be deleted.) If the database is large, packing data can take a long time.

packing data the deletion of vacant slots from a database.

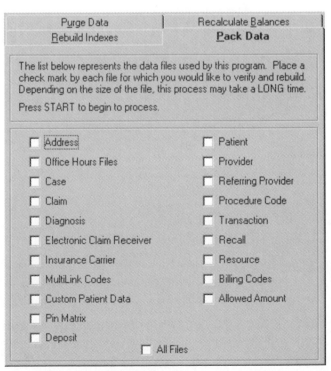

Figure 11-6 **Pack Data tab.**

To pack files in an office situation, you would complete the following steps.

1. Click File Maintenance on the File menu. The File Maintenance dialog box is displayed with the Rebuild Indexes tab active. Make the Pack Data tab active.

2. Click in each check box next to the files that are to have deleted data removed.

   If all files are to be checked for deleted data, click the All Files box at the bottom of the list of files.

3. Click the Start button. The Confirm dialog box is displayed with the message "All of the checked file processes will be performed. Do you want to continue?" Click the OK button to continue. (Clicking the Cancel button aborts the process.)

4. The pack process is performed automatically. When the process is complete, the message "All checked file processes are complete" is displayed.

Purging Data

purging data the process of deleting files of patients who are no longer seen by a provider in a practice.

The process of deleting files of patients who are no longer seen by a provider in a practice is called **purging data**. Purging data frees space on the computer and permits the system to run more efficiently. *However, purging should be done with great caution.* Once data is purged from the system, it cannot be retrieved, except from a backup file. As a safety precaution, always perform a backup before purging.

The Purge Data tab offers several options (see Figure 11-7). Data can be purged for appointments, claims, appointment recalls, audit data, or closed cases. All options except Purge Closed Cases are purged by date. A cutoff date is entered, and MediSoft deletes all data up to that date. For example, if all the data entered prior to December 31, 1994, are to be purged, that date would be entered as the cutoff date. Data entered in cases that have been closed are purged by clicking the check box labeled "Purge Closed Cases."

To purge data in an office situation, you would complete the following steps.

1. Click File Maintenance on the File menu. The File Maintenance dialog box is displayed with the Rebuild Indexes tab active. Make the Purge Data tab active.

2. Click in each check box next to the files that are to be purged. Enter a cutoff date in the Cutoff Dates box.

3. Click the Start button. The Confirm dialog box is displayed with the message "All of the checked file processes will be performed.

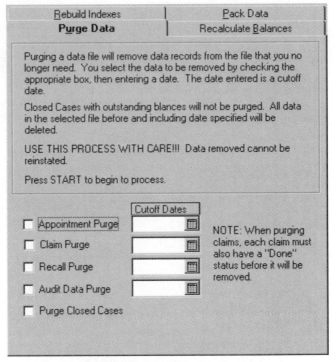

Figure 11-7 **Purge Data tab.**

Do you want to continue?" Click the OK button to continue. (Clicking the Cancel button aborts the process.)

4. The purge process is performed automatically. When the process is complete, the message "All checked file processes are complete" is displayed.

Recalculating Patient Balances

As transaction entries are changed or deleted, there are times when the balance listed on-screen is not accurate. To update balances to reflect the most recent changes made to the data, the Recalculate Balances feature is used. This feature is accessed through the Recalculate Balances tab on the File Maintenance dialog box (see Figure 11-8 on page 224).

When balances are recalculated, the system reviews every patient's data and recalculates the balances. The process of recalculating balances can be time-consuming. Individual patient balances can be recalculated in the Transaction Entry dialog box by clicking the Account Total column.

To recalculate balances in an office situation, you would complete the following steps.

1. Click File Maintenance on the File menu. The File Maintenance dialog box is displayed with the Rebuild Indexes tab active. Make the Recalculate Balances tab active.

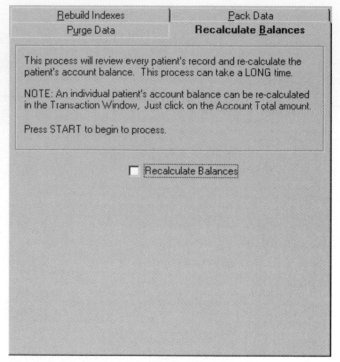

Figure 11-8 **Recalculate Balances tab.**

2. Click to place a check mark in the Recalculate Balances box.

3. Click the Start button. The Confirm dialog box is displayed with the message "All of the checked file processes will be performed. Do you want to continue?" Click the OK button to continue. (Clicking the Cancel button aborts the process.)

4. The recalculate process is performed automatically. When the process is complete, the message "All checked file processes are complete" is displayed.

USING TERMINOLOGY

Match the terms on the left with the definitions on the right.

_____ **1.** packing data

_____ **2.** purging data

_____ **3.** rebuilding indexes

_____ **4.** removable media device

_____ **5.** restoring data

a. A device that stores data but is not a permanent part of a computer.

b. A process that checks and verifies data and corrects any internal problems with the data.

c. The process of retrieving data from backup storage devices.

d. The deletion of vacant data slots from a database.

e. The process of deleting files of patients who are no longer seen by a provider of a practice.

CHECKING YOUR UNDERSTANDING

Answer the questions below in the space provided.

6. Why is it important to back up data regularly?

_____

_____

7. Why is extra caution required when purging data?

_____

_____

8. When is a data restore performed?

_____

_____

9. In MediSoft, where are the two places a patient's balance can be recalculated?

_____

_____

APPLYING KNOWLEDGE

Answer the question below in the space provided.

10. You come in to work on a Monday morning and find that the office computer is not working. The system manager informs everyone that the computer's hard disk crashed, and that all data that were not backed up are lost. What do you do?

_____

_____

_____

_____

Applying Your Knowledge

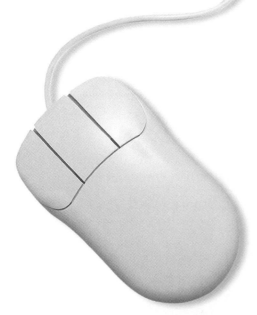

PART 3

CHAPTER

12

Handling Patient Records and Transactions

To complete the exercises in this chapter, you need to know how to:

◆ Locate patient information.

◆ Change the MediSoft Program Date.

◆ Assign a new chart number and enter information on a new patient.

◆ Create a new case for a patient.

◆ Change information on an established patient.

◆ Add an insurance company to the database.

◆ Enter procedures, charges, and diagnoses.

◆ Record payments from patients and insurance carriers.

◆ Print walkout receipts.

All office personnel at the Family Care Center (FCC) know how to input patient information in the Patient/Guarantor dialog box and in the Case dialog box. Whenever possible, all information for both dialog boxes is entered into the computer as soon as patients complete the handwritten information sheet and return it to the receptionist. On busy days, however, or when the office is understaffed because one of the medical assistants is sick or on vacation, input operations may be delayed.

EXERCISE 12-1: INPUTTING PATIENT INFORMATION

For this exercise, you need Source Documents 10–13.

It is Monday, November 15, 2004. You are a records/billing clerk at the Family Care Center. On your desk is a small pile of information sheets and superbills from Friday afternoon, November 12. You decide to input all patient information first, and then go back and record the transactions. First, you arrange the papers alphabetically:

Battistuta

Brooks

Hsu

Syzmanski

Then you begin. (Remember to change the MediSoft Program Date to November 15, 2004.)

Patient 1: Anthony Battistuta

Record the address and phone number changes that are written on Mr. Battistuta's superbill (Source Document 10).

1. Click Patients/Guarantors and Cases on the Lists menu. The Patient List dialog box is displayed.

2. Select Anthony Battistuta from the list of patients.

3. Click the Edit Patient button. The Patient/Guarantor dialog box is displayed, with the Name, Address tab active.

4. Enter the new address and phone number.

5. Click the Save button.

Patient 2: Lawana Brooks

You can see from the superbill (Source Document 11) that Ms. Brooks is an established patient. There are no changes to be made for her in the Patient/Guarantor dialog box. The work you need to do must take place in the Case dialog box. Ms. Brooks has had an accident at work, so a new case must be created.

1. After saving the changes for Mr. Battistuta in the Patient/ Guarantor dialog box, the Patient List dialog box is redisplayed.

2. In the list of patients, click the listing for Brooks to select her as the patient. In the list of cases, click the ankle sprain case. (You will not enter new information in the ankle sprain case; instead, you will copy information from the ankle sprain case to create a new case.)

3. Click the Copy Case button to copy the information from the existing case into a new case. A duplicate case is displayed.

4. Using Source Documents 11 and 12, edit the information in the case to reflect the information relevant to the new case by changing the information in the MediSoft boxes listed below. If a box is not listed, either the information in that box does not need to be changed, or the box is to remain blank.

Personal Tab

Description

Account Tab

Referring Provider: (delete existing entry)

Authorized Number of Visits: (delete existing entry)

ID: (delete existing entry)

Last Visit Date: (delete existing entry)

Last Visit Number: (delete existing entry)

Diagnosis Tab

Diagnosis 1

Diagnosis 2

Diagnosis 3

Condition Tab

Injury/Illness/LMP Date

Illness Indicator

First Consultation Date

Employment Related

Emergency

Accident Related to

Nature of

5. Save your work.

> **TIP▷** When entering information on different tabs within a dialog box, it is not necessary to click the Save button after completing each tab. However, the Save button must be clicked once all the tabs are complete, before exiting the dialog box.

Patient 3: Edwin Hsu

1. The information you need to make the necessary changes to the Patient/Guarantor dialog box for Edwin Hsu is on Source Documents 13 and 14. The new insurance company, Midwest Select, is not on the patient information form, nor is it in FCC's database. Edwin Hsu does not have his insurance card. You look up Midwest Select in the phone book, find the correct zip code on the map in the front of the phone book, and call the insurance company to find out what percentage of charges are covered by the plan. Midwest pays 80 percent after a $20 copayment.

2. After saving the new case for Brooks, you are in the Patient List dialog box. Select Edwin Hsu, and click the Edit Patient button.

3. Move to the Street box, and enter the new address.

4. Move to the Phones 1 box and enter the new phone number.

5. Save the information you just entered.

6. Now the new insurance carrier must be added to the database. From the Lists menu, click Insurance Carriers.

TIP▷ If the entire dialog box is not visible on your screen, resize the dialog box or use the scroll bars to see the additional entries.

7. The Insurance Carrier List dialog box is displayed.

8. Click the New Button to add information for Midwest Select.

9. Using the information on Source Document 14, enter the information in the following boxes.

   Address Tab

   Code

   Name

   Street

   City

   State

   Zip Code

   Phone

   Practice ID

Plan Name

Type

Procedure Code Set

Diagnosis Code Set

Signature on File

Default Billing Method

Print PINs on Forms

EMC Receiver

EMC Payor Number

EMC Sub ID

NDC Record Code

Payment

Adjustment

Notice that there is no adjustment code for Midwest Select, so one must be created.

With the Adjustment drop-down list visible, press the F8 key to display the Procedure/Payment/Adjustment: (new) dialog box.

In the Code 1 box, key *MIDADJ*. Press the Tab key once.

Key *Midwest Select Adjustment* in the Description box. Press the Tab key.

Accept the default entries in the other boxes.

Since this is an adjustment entry, no entries need to be made in the Amounts and Allowed Amounts tabs.

Click the Save button. The Procedure/Payment/Adjustment dialog box closes and MIDADJ is displayed in the Adjustment box on the EMC, Codes tab for Midwest Select.

Since this is a capitated HMO, there is no deductible, so the Deductible box should be left blank.

10. Click the Save button. Midwest Select is now displayed on the list of insurance carriers.

11. With Midwest Select highlighted, click the Edit button. Using Source Document 14, complete the following boxes in the PINs tab.

Provider   PIN   Group ID

McGrath

Beach

Banu

12. Click the Save button.

13. Close the Insurance Carrier List dialog box. The Patient List dialog box is still displayed. Edwin Hsu is still the selected patient.

14. Create a new case for Edwin Hsu by copying his existing case.

15. Using Source Documents 13 and 14, edit the information in the copied case to reflect the information relevant to the new case. Change information in the following boxes:

Personal Tab

Description

Account Tab

Price Code

Diagnosis Tab

Diagnosis 1

Condition Tab

Injury/Illness/LMP Date

Illness Indicator

Policy 1 Tab

Insurance 1

Policy Number

Group Number

Policy Dates Start

Capitated Plan

Copayment Amount

Insurance Coverage Percents by Service Classification: Enter 80 in all boxes

16. Click the Save button to save the new case.

> **TIP** ▷ Do not change the insurance carrier in the urinary tract infection case for Edwin Hsu, because at the time he was treated for that condition, Hsu was covered by East Ohio PPO, not Midwest Select.

Patient 4: Hannah Syzmanski

Use Source Documents 15 and 16 to enter information on a new patient, Hannah Syzmanski. Hannah is the daughter of Michael and Debra Syzmanski, who are patients of Dr. Dana Banu. Hannah has been seeing her own doctor, a pediatrician, but is now switching to the Family Care Center.

1. Go to the Patient List dialog box, and click the New Patient button.

2. Key *SYZMAHA0* in the Chart Number box.

3. Complete the boxes for name, address, phone, birth date, sex, and Social Security number.

4. Complete the following boxes in the Other Information tab.

   Type

   Assigned Provider

   Signature on File

   Signature Date

5. Save your work.

6. Click the Case radio button to make the Case portion of the Patient List dialog box active.

7. Click the New Case button to open a new Case dialog box.

8. Complete the following tabs in the Case dialog box.

   Personal Tab

   Description

   Guarantor

   Marital Status

   Student Status

   Account Tab

   Referring Provider

   Price Code: B

Diagnosis Tab

Diagnosis 1

Allergies and Notes

Policy 1 Tab

When you attempt to complete the Policy 1 tab, you notice that Hannah has not filled in her insurance company, but since she is covered by her father's insurance, you know that information will be easy to find if necessary.

First save your work on Hannah's case. Then open the Case dialog box for the acne case for Michael Syzmanski, and go to the Policy 1 tab. Use the information on that tab to fill in the missing insurance data for Hannah Syzmanski.

When completing the Policy 1 tab for Hannah, remember to list Michael Syzmanski in the Policy Holder 1 box and to click Child in the Relationship to Insured field.

9. Save your work.

EXERCISE 12-2: AN EMERGENCY VISIT

You will need Source Document 17 for this exercise.

It is still Monday morning, November 15, 2004. Carlos Lopez has just seen Dr. McGrath on an emergency basis. Mr. Lopez thought he was having a heart attack. Fortunately, Dr. McGrath has determined that he was just suffering from heart palpitations. You need to enter the procedure charges, accept his payment, and print a walkout receipt. Make sure all transaction information is properly recorded in the database.

1. Verify that the MediSoft Program Date is November 15, 2004.

2. From the Patient List dialog box, create a new case for Carlos Lopez by copying the information in the case that already exists.

3. Using Source Document 17, complete the following boxes.

Personal Tab

Description

Diagnosis Tab

Diagnosis 1

Condition Tab

Injury/Illness/LMP Date

Illness Indicator

First Consultation Date

Emergency

4. Save your work.

5. Click Enter Transactions on the Activities menu.

6. Select Mr. Lopez in the Chart box.

7. Select heart palpitations in the Case box.

8. Click the New button to create a new transaction. The Charge tab is active.

9. If necessary, key *11152004* in both Dates boxes.

10. If necessary, change the date in the Document box to 0411150000.

11. Enter the first procedure number checked on the superbill.

12. Save the transaction and open a new transaction by clicking the Save/Open button. A dialog box opens with the reminder that the case requires a $15.00 copay. Click the OK button to close the dialog box.

13. Enter the other procedure number from the superbill.

14. Click the Save/Open button to save the transaction. Now enter Lopez's copayment and apply the payment to the charges.

    Hint: In the Pay Code box, select the option that reads "OHC-COPAY—OhioCare HMO Copayment."

15. Click the Save/Close button to save the transaction and return to the Transaction Entry dialog box.

16. Click the Print Receipt button to print a walkout receipt.

EXERCISE 12-3: INPUTTING TRANSACTION DATA

For this exercise, you need Source Documents 10, 11, 13, and 16.

You are now ready to record the transactions from Friday's four superbills. Before you begin, set the MediSoft Program Date to November 12, 2004.

Anthony Battistuta

1. Click Enter Transactions on the Activities menu.

2. Select Anthony Battistuta in the Chart box.

3. Verify that Diabetes is displayed to the right of the Case box.

4. Record the procedures, one at a time.

5. Save your work.

Lawana Brooks

Follow essentially the same procedures to enter the transaction data. Remember to save your work.

Edwin Hsu

Follow essentially the same procedures to enter the transaction data. You need to record the date and procedure, and Hsu's payment. Apply the payment to the charges, and save your work.

Hannah Syzmanski

Follow essentially the same procedures to enter the transaction data. You need to record the date and procedure, and Syzmanski's payment. Apply the payment to the charges, and save your work.

EXERCISE 12-4: ENTERING A NEW PATIENT AND TRANSACTIONS

For this exercise, you need Source Documents 18 and 19.

The date is November 12, 2004. Enter patient information and all transactions for Christopher Palmer, a new patient of Dr. Beach.

EXERCISE 12-5: ENTERING AND APPLYING AN INSURANCE CARRIER PAYMENT

For this exercise, you need Source Document 20.

The date is November 12, 2004. A remittance advice has just been received from East Ohio PPO with a check attached. Enter the deposit in MediSoft and apply the payment to the appropriate patient accounts.

1. Open the Deposit List dialog box.

2. Change the date in the Deposit Date box to November 12, 2004.

3. Enter the deposit.

4. Apply the payment to the patient charges. Be sure to click the Save Payments/Adjustments button after each patient. Notice that as you enter and save payments, the amount listed in the Unapplied box decreases.

5. When you are finished, verify that the amount in the Unapplied column in the Deposit List dialog box for the deposit on 11/12/2004 is 0.00.

6. Payments entered in the Deposit List dialog box are automatically linked to data in the Transaction Entry dialog box. Open the Transaction Entry dialog box and confirm that the insurance company payments and adjustments appear in the transaction list at the bottom of the window for each patient in this exercise.

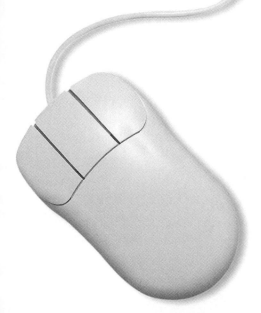

CHAPTER

13

Setting Up Appointments

WHAT YOU NEED TO KNOW

To complete the exercises in this chapter, you need to know how to:

◆ Start Office Hours.

◆ Move around in the schedule.

◆ Enter appointments.

◆ Change appointment information.

◆ Move or copy an appointment.

◆ Schedule a recall appointment.

◆ Create a new case record for a patient.

◆ Change a transaction record.

The Family Care Center uses Office Hours as the primary tool for recording appointments. For the simulations in this chapter, assume that you are the front-desk receptionist/clerk and are responsible for most of the Center's scheduling tasks. Remember, you can access Office Hours at any time, no matter what you are working on. For example, suppose you are typing a letter for one of the doctors, and you get a phone call from a patient who wants to make an appointment. All you have to do is click the Start button on the task bar; select Programs—MediSoft, and then Office Hours; enter the appointment; exit Office Hours; and return to your word processing program. Office Hours can also be accessed from within MediSoft, either by clicking the shortcut button or by clicking Appointment Book on the Activities menu.

EXERCISE 13-1 SCHEDULING APPOINTMENTS

It is Monday, November 15, 2004. In Office Hours, schedule the following patient appointments on December 10, 2004:

Patient	Provider	Time	Length
Nancy Stern	P. McGrath	9:30	30 minutes
Sheila Giles	R. Beach	10:00	45 minutes
Raji Patel	D. Banu	2:45	30 minutes

1. Open Office Hours.

2. Go to December 10, 2004.

3. Select each patient's provider from the Provider drop-down list and enter the appointments.

EXERCISE 13-2: MAKING AN APPOINTMENT CHANGE

Carlos Lopez has just called to say that he has lost his appointment card and cannot remember what time his appointment is on December 1. He thinks there may be a scheduling conflict with a meeting he has that day. If the appointment is in the morning, he wants you to change it to 2:00 p.m. that same day. If the 2:00 p.m. slot is not available, he needs to make the appointment for the next day at the earliest possible time.

1. Open Office Hours if it is not already open.

2. Go to December 1, 2004.

3. Find out who Lopez's doctor is by calling up the Patient/Guarantor dialog box in MediSoft. Select the Other Information tab, and check the Assigned Provider box. Then select Lopez's provider from the Provider drop-down list in Office Hours.

4. Locate Mr. Lopez's appointment.

5. Check to see whether 2:00 p.m., the time he wanted to change the appointment to, is available.

6. Since 2:00 is not available, move to December 2 on the calendar and see if 8:00 a.m. is available.

7. Go back to December 1. Move Mr. Lopez's appointment from December 1 to December 2. (If you do not remember how to move an appointment, see Chapter 8.)

EXERCISE 13-3: JUGGLING SCHEDULES

Mrs. Jackson's sister is on the phone. She will be taking care of the Jackson twins, Darnell and Tyrone, on Saturday, December 11, 2004, and she needs to make an appointment for both of them for physicals and tetanus shots sometime after 9:00 a.m. That is the only day they can come in, so she hopes you can accommodate her. She does not remember the name of their doctor.

1. Find out who the twins' doctor is by looking up the information in MediSoft.

2. Go into Office Hours, and check the twin's provider's schedule for December 11. She is booked solid from 9:00 a.m. until she leaves at 1:00 p.m.

3. Check the schedules of Dr. McGrath and Dr. Beach. Since Dr. McGrath is unavailable, book Darnell in the 10:30 a.m. time slot and Tyrone in the 10:45 a.m. slot with Dr. Beach.

EXERCISE 13-4: ADDING PATIENTS TO THE RECALL LIST

Darnell and Tyrone Jackson need to be called back for follow-up appointments in six months. Add both of them to the Recall list for six months from December 11, 2004.

1. Click Patient Recall on the Lists menu (in MediSoft). The Patient Recall List dialog box is displayed.

2. Click the New button.

3. Enter June 11, 2005, in the Recall Date box.

4. Select Dr. Dana Banu in the Provider box.

5. Key the first six letters of Darnell Jackson's chart number in the Chart box. Press the Tab key.

6. In the Message box, key *Six month follow-up appointment needed.*

7. Verify that the Call radio button in the Recall Status box is selected.

8. Click the Save button to save the entry.

9. Repeat the steps to add Tyrone Jackson to the Patient Recall List.

10. Close the Patient Recall List dialog box.

EXERCISE 13-5: DIANE HSU AND MICHAEL SYZMANSKI

For this simulation, you will need Source Documents 21 and 22.

It is Monday, November 15, 2004. Diane Hsu and Michael Syzman-ski are leaving the office after their appointments. Use the information on Source Documents 21 and 22 to perform the following tasks:

1. Create new cases for both patients by copying existing cases.

   For Hsu, complete the boxes listed below in the Personal, Account, Diagnosis, and Policy 1 tabs. When completing the Account and Policy 1 tabs for Hsu, remember that her husband changed insurance carriers to Midwest Select, and since she is covered under her husband's policy, the new insurance company information must be used. This information can be found in Edwin Hsu's acute sinusitis case (see also Source Document 14).

   Personal Tab

   Description

   Account Tab

   Price Code

   Diagnosis Tab

   Diagnosis 1

   Policy 1 Tab

   Insurance 1

   Policy Number

   Group Number

   Policy Dates Start

   Capitated Plan

   Copayment Amount

   Insurance Coverage Percents by Service Classification

   For Syzmanski, complete the following boxes in the Personal and Diagnosis tabs.

   Personal Tab

   Description

   Diagnosis Tab

   Diagnosis 1

2. Record the charges in the Transaction Entry dialog box.

3. Record the payments and apply the payments to the charges.

4. Print walkout receipts.

5. Make the appointment indicated on Mrs. Hsu's superbill, using Office Hours. Do not exit MediSoft.

EXERCISE 13-6: CHANGING A TRANSACTION RECORD

Just as you finish making Mrs. Hsu's appointment, Dr. Robert Beach comes to the desk to say that he thinks he forgot to put down on the superbill the strep test he performed on Christopher Palmer on November 12, 2004. He asks you to check and add the charge if necessary.

1. Go to the Transaction Entry dialog box. Check through the entries to find out whether the charge was entered. (It was not.)

2. Enter the new charge. (Hint: Remember to change the default date entries in the Dates boxes to November 12, 2004.)

3. Save your work.

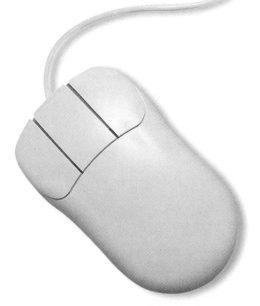

CHAPTER

14

Printing Lists and Reports

WHAT YOU NEED TO KNOW

To complete the exercises in this chapter, you need to know how to:

◆ Create a patient ledger.
◆ Create a day sheet report.
◆ Understand what aging means, in an accounting sense.
◆ Create a patient aging report.
◆ Enter transactions.
◆ Print an appointment list.
◆ Print a patient ledger report.

Because MediSoft is an accounting package, its most powerful features involve computerized manipulation of account data for patients. MediSoft uses information in the system to produce reports on any facet of patients' or insurers' accounts and to generate bills for patients and insurance companies. For example, as long as the office personnel in the Family Care Center have entered transactions correctly and have performed basic accounting procedures, the MediSoft program can be used to print current reports on the center's finances. You can print a report showing details of a day's transactions for any one of the center's physicians or for all physicians. You can print a report of late accounts for a particular patient, for all patients, for one insurance company, or for all insurance companies.

Before starting the exercises in this chapter, you should understand some basic aspects of medical office accounting procedures.

Every medical office must keep a daily record of charges and payments made for every patient of every doctor. For charges, the record usually includes the name of the patient, the type of service provided, and the amount of the charge. For payments, the record usually includes the name of the patient whose account is being credited and the amount of the payment. Whereas day sheets record information on charges and payments for a single day, ledgers show all current information up to and including the date shown on the ledger.

As the name suggests, aging reports show clearly how long unpaid charges have been due. In MediSoft, aging reports are divided into four columns, showing, in order, accounts that are currently due, accounts that have been due for 31–60 days, accounts that have been due for 61–90 days, and accounts that have been due for more than 90 days.

EXERCISE 14-1: FINDING A PATIENT'S BALANCE

It is still Monday, November 15, 2004. Anthony Battistuta calls. He would like to know the amount of the charges from November 12 that he is responsible for, assuming Medicare pays its portion of the total charges. How can you find the amount he is responsible for?

MediSoft Program Date: November 15, 2004

1. On the Activities menu, click Enter Transactions.

2. In the Chart box, select Anthony Battistuta's chart number.

3. Verify that the Diabetes case is active in the Case box.

4. Look at the left side of the dialog box, where the information about financial responsibility is listed. Determine the insurance carrier's portion of the charges, and then determine what amount of the charges is the guarantor's responsibility.

EXERCISE 14-2: PRINTING A SCHEDULE

Print the appointment schedule for Dr. Dana Banu for Saturday, December 11, 2004.

1. Open Office Hours.

2. Select Dr. Dana Banu as the Provider.

3. Go to December 11, 2004 in the calendar.

4. Click Appointment List on the Office Hours Reports menu.

5. Select the option to print the report on the printer.

6. Click the Start button.

7. Exit Office Hours

EXERCISE 14-3: PRINTING DAY SHEET REPORTS

Patient day sheets and procedure day sheets can be viewed and/or printed using options on the Reports menu.

MediSoft Program Date: November 12, 2004

Creating a Patient Day Sheet Report

1. On the Reports menu, click Day Sheets and then Patient Day Sheet.

2. Select the option to preview the report on-screen. Click the Start button.

3. Leave the Chart Number Range boxes blank, to include all patients.

4. Delete the entries in both of the Date Created Range boxes.

5. Key *11122004* in both of Date From Range boxes.

6. Leave all the other boxes blank.

7. Click the OK button.

8. The patient day sheet report is displayed on-screen.

9. Close the Preview Report window.

Creating a Procedure Day Sheet Report

1. On the Reports menu, click Day Sheets and then Procedure Day Sheet.

2. Select the option to preview the report on-screen. Click the Start button.

3. Leave the Procedure Code Range boxes blank.

4. Delete both entries in the Date Created Range boxes.

5. Key *11122004* in both of the Date From Range boxes.

6. Leave the Attending Provider boxes blank.

7. Click the OK button.

8. The procedure day sheet report appears on-screen.

9. Close the Preview Report window.

EXERCISE 14-4: CREATING A PATIENT AGING REPORT

Print a patient aging report as a first step in the billing process. The aging report shows which accounts are overdue and how long they have been overdue.

MediSoft Program Date: December 31, 2004

1. On the Reports menu, click Aging Reports and then Patient Aging.

2. Select the option to preview the report on-screen. Click the Start button.

3. Leave all data selection fields blank except the second Date From Range box. Key *12312004* in this box.

4. Click the OK button.

5. View the report.

6. Close the Preview Report window.

EXERCISE 14-5: STEWART ROBERTSON

You need Source Document 23 and 24 for this exercise, which consists of two parts. For the first part, assume that it is December 10, 2004. A new patient of Dr. Beach, Stewart Robertson, has stopped by to fill out a patient information form, and he wants an appointment for December, specifically for the third Saturday of the month, as early as possible. He needs an appointment for a routine physical.

Part One - December 10, 2004
MediSoft Program Date: December 10, 2004

1. Using Source Document 23, enter the patient information for Mr. Robertson. Complete the Patient/Guarantor dialog box and the Case dialog box. You need to create a new case.

2. In Office Hours, schedule Robertson for his appointment.

Part Two - December 18, 2004
MediSoft Program Date: December 18, 2004

1. Using Source Document 24, enter Robertson's diagnosis in MediSoft.

2. Enter the charges and payments for Stewart Robertson's visit.

3. Print a walkout receipt for Mr. Robertson.

EXERCISE 14-6: MICHAEL SYZMANSKI

MediSoft Program Date: December 18, 2004

1. Read the following account of Michael Syzmanski's visit to the Family Care Center on December 18, 2004.

   While driving to his daughter Hannah's soccer game, Syzmanski had a minor automobile accident in Jefferson and has a cut on his eyelid. He has come in to see Dr. Banu on an emergency basis. Dr. Banu is unavailable, so he is treated by Dr. McGrath. She determines that there has been no serious damage. After an examination using a local anesthetic, Dr. McGrath stitches the cut and tells Syzmanski to come back in a week. The procedure is simple suture with local anesthesia.

2. In MediSoft, enter all the information pertaining to this visit using Source Document 25.

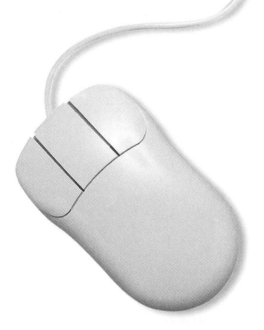

Printing Statements and Creating Claims

WHAT YOU NEED TO KNOW

To complete the exercises in this chapter, you need to know how to:

◆ Print patient statements.

◆ Create insurance claims.

◆ Print insurance claim forms.

Different medical practices have different billing procedures. The Family Care Center collects copayments from patients at the time service is rendered. The center then bills the insurance company. Once a remittance advice is received from the carrier, the patient is billed for the remainder. Bills for remainder balances are mailed out on the fifteenth of the month for patients whose last names begin with A–L and on the thirtieth of the month for patients whose last names begin with M–Z.

EXERCISE 15-1: PRINTING PATIENT STATEMENTS

Today's date is December 18, 2004. Michael Syzmanski would like a copy of his patient statement before he leaves the office (Exercise 14-6).

MediSoft Program Date: December 18, 2004

1. Click Patient Statements on the Reports menu.

2. Click Patient Statement (30, 60, 90) in the Open Report dialog box.

3. Click the appropriate radio button to preview the statement on-screen. Click the Start button.

4. Enter Syzmanski's chart number in both Chart Number Range boxes.

5. Enter December 18, 2004, in the second Date From Range box. Leave the first Date From Range box and the other data selection boxes blank.

6. Click the OK button.

7. Preview the statement. Notice that because Michael is guarantor on his daughter Hannah's account, her charges appear on his statement.

8. Print the statement.

9. Close the Preview Report window.

EXERCISE 15-2: CREATING INSURANCE CLAIMS

Create insurance claims for patients who have had transactions from November 12, 2004, to November 30, 2004.

MediSoft Program Date: November 30, 2004

1. Click Claim Management on the Activities menu.

2. Click the Create Claims button.

3. Key *11122004* in the first Transaction Dates box and *11302004* in the second.

4. Leave the rest of the boxes blank.

5. Click the Create button.

6. The new claims are recorded at the end of the list in the Claim Management dialog box.

7. Do not exit the Claim Management dialog box.

EXERCISE 15-3: PRINTING INSURANCE CLAIM FORMS

Print an insurance claim form for Carlos Lopez.

MediSoft Program Date: November 30, 2004

1. In the Claim Management dialog box, select Lopez's claim.

2. Click the Edit button.

3. For the purposes of this exercise, change the Billing Method from Electronic to Paper. Click the Save button.

4. Click the Print/Send button.

5. Click the Paper radio button to select claims with a default billing method of paper, if it is not already selected.

6. Click the OK button.

7. Select HCFA 1500 (Primary) from the list of reports in the Open Report dialog box. Click the OK button.

8. Select the option to preview the form on-screen. Click the Start button.

9. Enter Lopez's chart number in both Chart Number Range boxes.

10. Click the OK button.

11. Preview the form on-screen, and then print it.

12. Close the Preview Report window.

13. Close the Claim Management dialog box.

EXERCISE 15-4: PRINTING REMAINDER STATEMENTS FOR PATIENTS WITH OUTSTANDING BALANCES

MediSoft Program Date: November 30, 2004

Print remainder statements for all patients whose last names begin with the letters A through L and who have outstanding balances as of November 30, 2004. Figure 15-1 on page 256 shows the Open Report dialog box with the appropriate report highlighted. Figure 15-2 on the same page shows the Data Selection Questions dialog box for this task.

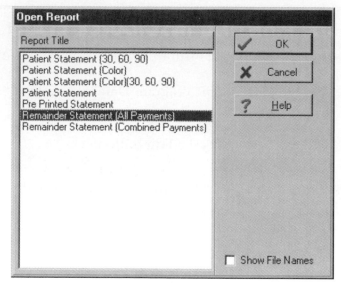

Figure 15-1 **Open Report dialog box.**

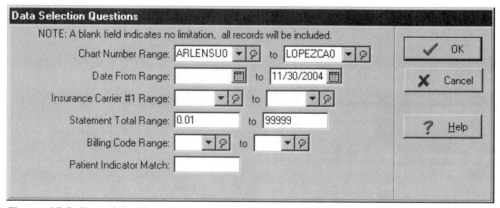

Figure 15-2 **Data Selection Questions dialog box.**

EXERCISE 15-5: VIEWING CLAIMS FOR PATIENTS WITH MEDICARE AS THEIR PRIMARY INSURANCE CARRIER

MediSoft Program Date: November 30, 2004

1. Display insurance claims for all patients who have Medicare as their primary insurance carrier. Figure 15-3 shows the List Only Claims That Match dialog box for this task.

2. Use the Edit feature to review the transaction information contained in Randall Klein's claim.

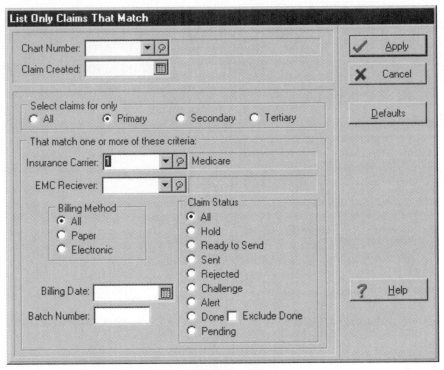

Figure 15-3 **List Only Claims That Match dialog box.**

EXERCISE 15-6: PUTTING IT ALL TOGETHER

For this exercise, you need to use almost all the skills you have practiced in the preceding material.

1. Enter January 5, 2005, as the program date in MediSoft.

2. Schedule appointments for January 5, 2005, for the following patients. Make sure they are scheduled for the right doctors.

Jackson, Luther	30 minutes	9:00 a.m.
Hsu, Diane	15 minutes	9:00 a.m.
Hsu, Edwin	15 minutes	9:15 a.m.
Simmons, Jill	15 minutes	9:00 a.m.
Stern, Nancy	1 hour	9:30 a.m.
Syzmanski, Debra	30 minutes	9:30 a.m.
Giles, Sheila	15 minutes	10:15 a.m.
Battistuta, Pauline	30 minutes	10:30 a.m.

3. Switch the appointment times for Giles and Simmons.

4. Cancel both of the Hsus' appointments.

5. Print the appointment lists for January 5, 2005, for Dr. Banu, Dr. Beach, and Dr. McGrath.

6. Create new cases for all patients with appointments on January 5, 2005. Fill in the following boxes on the Personal and Diagnosis tabs using the information found on Source Documents 26–31.

Personal Tab

Description

Diagnosis Tab

Diagnosis 1

7. Using Source Documents 26–31, record the charge and payment transactions for each of the patients who had appointments. Be sure to save each of these transactions before you proceed to the next one. Print walkout receipts for patients who made payments.

8. Print patient day sheets for all the patients with transactions on January 5, 2005.

9. Create insurance claims for the day's transactions.

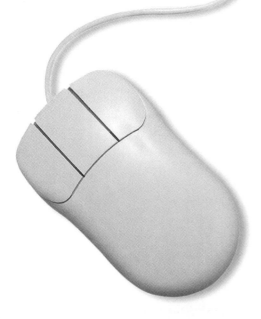

16 Filing Electronic Media Claims

WHAT YOU NEED TO KNOW

To complete the exercises in this chapter, you need to know how to:

◆ Create electronic claims.

◆ Send claims electronically to insurance carriers.

◆ Review an audit/edit report.

◆ Review claims for errors and omissions.

ELECTRONIC CLAIM REQUIREMENTS

Insurance carriers use different claim formats when processing electronic claims. For this reason, many medical offices send their electronic claims to a clearinghouse, which checks the data and translates it into the appropriate format for the particular carrier. The clearinghouse then sends the claim to the insurance carrier.

As the largest processor of health insurance claims in the United States, Medicare is also the industry's leader in processing electronic claims. More than 80 percent of Medicare Part B claims from participating physicians are processed electronically. In the near future, all Medicare- and Medicaid-participating providers will be required to submit their claims electronically.

Medicare requires that certain boxes be filled in on electronic claims. These are known as mandatory boxes. Other boxes are conditional; that is, whether they need to be filled in depends on other information. For example, the name of a patient's employer is a conditional box; it needs to be completed only if a patient is employed. The following table lists each box that must be filled in when submitting electronic claims to Medicare, and its corresponding location in MediSoft.

Table 16-1   Medicare Mandatory Boxes for Submitting Electronic Claims

Required Information	Dialog Box	Tab	Box
Insured's ID number	Case	Policy 1	Policy Number
Patient's name	Patient/Guarantor	Name, Address	Last Name First Name
Insured's policy group number	Case	Policy 1	Group Number
Patient's signature source	Patient/Guarantor	Other Information	Signature on File
Dates of service	Transaction Entry	Charge	Dates
Place of service	Transaction Entry	Charge	POS
Procedures	Transaction Entry	Charge	Procedure
Charges	Transaction Entry	Charge	Amount
Units of service	Transaction Entry	Charge	Units
Provider's signature indicator	Provider	Address	Signature on File
Provider's billing name and address	Provider	Address	Last Name First Name
Payer organization	Practice Information		Practice Name
Provider Medicare Number	Provider	PINs	Medicare PIN
Provider's pay to address	Provider	Address	Street
Provider's pay to city	Provider	Address	City
Provider's pay to state	Provider	Address	State
Provider's pay to Zip Code	Provider	Address	Zip Code
Provider's pay to phone number	Provider	Address	Phone

EXERCISE 16-1: PERFORMING AN ON-SCREEN EDIT CHECK

Anthony Battistuta was seen by Dr. McGrath on November 12, 2004. Several charges have been entered, and an insurance claim has been created. Using the Medicare mandatory box guidelines, check to be certain that all the mandatory boxes are complete for the transactions on this claim. Make a list of any required boxes that are not complete.

EXERCISE 16-2: PREPARING A CLAIM FOR ELECTRONIC TRANSMISSION

Once data have been checked for accuracy and completeness, a claim is ready to be transmitted to the clearinghouse. While it is not possible to actually send claims in this simulation, they can be prepared for transmission. Perform all the steps necessary to submit Mr. Battistuta's claim for electronic transmission to a clearinghouse. When the Send Electronic Claims dialog box is displayed, do not click the Send Claims Now button. Because you are in a school setting and are not set up to submit electronic claims, click the Close button.

Source Documents

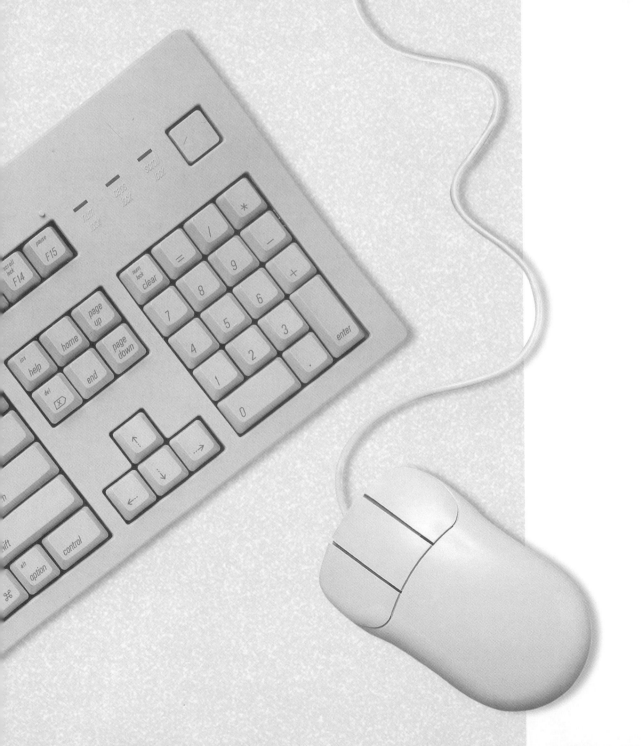

PATIENT INFORMATION FORM

THIS SECTION REFERS TO PATIENT ONLY

Name: Hiro Tanaka	Sex: F	Marital status: ☒S ☐M ☐D ☐W	Birth date: 2/20/75

Address: 80 Cedar Lane	SS#: 812-73-6000

City: Stephenson	State: OH	Zip: 60089	Employer: McCray Manufacturing Inc.

Home phone: 614-555-7373	Employer's address: 1311 Kings Highway

Work phone: 614-555-1001	City: Stephenson	State: OH	Zip: 60089

Spouse's name:	Spouse's employer:

Emergency contact:	Relationship:	Phone #:

FILL IN IF PATIENT IS A MINOR

Parent/Guardian's name:	Sex:	Marital status: ☐S ☐M ☐D ☐W	Birth date:

Phone:	SS#:

Address:	

City:	State:	Zip:	Employer:

Student status:	City:	State:	Zip:

INSURANCE INFORMATION

Primary insurance company: OhioCare HMO	Secondary insurance company:

Policyholder's name: Hiro Tanaka	Birth date: 2/20/75	Policyholder's name:	Birth date:

Copayment: $15	Price Code: A	Copayment:	Price Code:

Policy #: 812736000	Group #: HJ31	Policy #:	Group #:

OTHER INFORMATION

Reason for visit: Accident — back pain	Allergy to medication (list): penicillin

Name of referring physician: Dr. Bertram Brown	If auto accident, list date and state in which it occurred: 9/26/04 OH

Hiro Tanaka _____   10/4/2004 _____

(Patient's signature/Parent or guardian's signature)   (Date)

Family Care Center
285 Stephenson Boulevard
Stephenson, OH 60089
(614)555-0000

Date: 10/4/2004   **Name** Hiro Tanaka

Chart Number TANAKHIO   **Physician** Dr. Katherine Yan

01	patient payment, cash	85651	erythrocyte sedimentation rate--non-auto
02	patient payment, check	86403	strep test, quick
03	insurance carrier payment	86585	tuberculosis, tine test
04	insurance company adjustment	86588	direct streptococcus screen
05	adjustment, patient	87072	culture by commercial kit, nonurine...
12011	simple suture--face--local anes.	87076	bacterial culture, anerobic, with GC...
29125	application of short arm splint; static	87086	urine culture and colony count
29425	application of short leg cast, walking	90703	tetanus injection
45378	colonoscopy--diagnostic	90782	injection with material, subcutaneous or
45380	colonoscopy--with biopsy	92516	facial nerve function studies
50390	aspiration of renal cyst by needle	93000	Electrocardiogram--ECG with interpret...
71010	chest x-ray, single view, frontal	93015	Treadmill stress test, with physician...
71020	chest x-ray, two views, frontal & lat...	96900	ultraviolet light treatment
71030	chest x-ray, complete, four views	99070	supplies and materials provided
73070	elbow x-ray, AP and lateral views	99201	OF--new patient, problem focused
73090	forearm x-ray, AP and lateral views	99202	OF--new patient, expanded
73100	wrist x-ray, AP and lateral views	99203	OF--new patient, detailed history and...
73510	hip x-ray, complete, two views	99204	OF--new patient, comprehensive history..
73600	ankle x-ray, AP and lateral views	99205	OF--new patient, comprehensive history..
80019	19 clinical chemistry tests	99211	OF--established patient, minimal
80061	lipid panel	99212	OF--established patient, problem focused
82270	blood screening, occult; feces	99213	OF--established patient, expanded
82947	glucose screening--quantitative	99214	OF--established patient, detailed...
82951	glucose tolerance test, three specimens	99215	OF--established patient, comprehensive..
83718	HDL cholesterol	99394	established patient, adolescent, per...
84478	triglycerides test	99396	established patient, 40-64 years, per...
85007	manual differential WBC		
85022	hemogram, automated, and manual...		

Payments $15 copay, check #123   **Remarks**

Diagnosis 724.2

Physician's Notes for Hiro Takana
Date: 10/4/04

Case: Accident — back pain

Condition related to auto accident in Stephenson, Ohio that occurred on 9/26/04.

Hospitalized from 9/26/04 to 9/27/04.

Totally disabled from 9/26/04 to 9/27/04.

Partially disabled from 9/28/04 to 10/4/04.

Unable to work from 9/26/04 to 10/04/04.

Family Care Center
285 Stephenson Boulevard
Stephenson, OH 60089
(614)555-0000

Date: 10/4/2004

Name Elizabeth Jones

Chart Number JONESEL0

Physician Dr. Katherine Yan

01	patient payment, cash	85651	erythrocyte sedimentation rate--non-auto
02	patient payment, check	86403	strep test, quick
03	insurance carrier payment	86585	tuberculosis, tine test
04	insurance company adjustment	86588	direct streptococcus screen
05	adjustment, patient	87072	culture by commercial kit, nonurine...
12011	simple suture--face--local anes.	87076	bacterial culture, anerobic, with GC...
29125	application of short arm splint; static	87086	urine culture and colony count
29425	application of short leg cast, walking	90703	tetanus injection
45378	colonoscopy--diagnostic	90782	injection with material, subcutaneous or
45380	colonoscopy--with biopsy	92516	facial nerve function studies
50390	aspiration of renal cyst by needle	93000	Electrocardiogram--ECG with interpret...
71010	chest x-ray, single view, frontal	93015	Treadmill stress test, with physician...
71020	chest x-ray, two views, frontal & lat...	96900	ultraviolet light treatment
71030	chest x-ray, complete, four views	99070	supplies and materials provided
73070	elbow x-ray, AP and lateral views	99201	OF--new patient, problem focused
73090	forearm x-ray, AP and lateral views	99202	OF--new patient, expanded
73100	wrist x-ray, AP and lateral views	99203	OF--new patient, detailed history and...
73510	hip x-ray, complete, two views	99204	OF--new patient, comprehensive history..
73600	ankle x-ray, AP and lateral views	99205	OF--new patient, comprehensive history..
80019	19 clinical chemistry tests	99211	OF--established patient, minimal
80061	lipid panel	99212	OF--established patient, problem focused
82270	blood screening, occult; feces	99213	OF--established patient, expanded
82947	glucose screening--quantitative	99214	OF--established patient, detailed...
82951	glucose tolerance test, three specimens	99215	OF--established patient, comprehensive..
83718	HDL cholesterol	99394	established patient, adolescent, per...
84478	triglycerides test	99396	established patient, 40-64 years, per...
85007	manual differential WBC		
85022	hemogram, automated, and manual...		

Payments _____

Remarks _____

Diagnosis 250.0

Family Care Center
285 Stephenson Boulevard
Stephenson, OH 60089
(614)555-0000

Date: 10/4/2004   **Name** John Fitzwilliams

Chart Number FITZWJOO   **Physician** Dr. John Rudner

01	patient payment, cash		85651	erythrocyte sedimentation rate--non-auto
02	patient payment, check		86403	strep test, quick
03	insurance carrier payment		86585	tuberculosis, tine test
04	insurance company adjustment		86588	direct streptococcus screen
05	adjustment, patient		87072	culture by commercial kit, nonurine...
12011	simple suture--face--local anes.		87076	bacterial culture, anerobic, with GC...
29125	application of short arm splint; static		87086	urine culture and colony count
29425	application of short leg cast, walking		90703	tetanus injection
45378	colonoscopy--diagnostic		90782	injection with material, subcutaneous or
45380	colonoscopy--with biopsy		92516	facial nerve function studies
50390	aspiration of renal cyst by needle		93000	Electrocardiogram--ECG with interpret...
71010	chest x-ray, single view, frontal		93015	Treadmill stress test, with physician...
71020	chest x-ray, two views, frontal & lat...		96900	ultraviolet light treatment
71030	chest x-ray, complete, four views		99070	supplies and materials provided
73070	elbow x-ray, AP and lateral views		99201	OF--new patient, problem focused
73090	forearm x-ray, AP and lateral views		99202	OF--new patient, expanded
73100	wrist x-ray, AP and lateral views		99203	OF--new patient, detailed history and...
73510	hip x-ray, complete, two views		99204	OF--new patient, comprehensive history..
73600	ankle x-ray, AP and lateral views		99205	OF--new patient, comprehensive history..
80019	19 clinical chemistry tests		99211	OF--established patient, minimal
80061	lipid panel		99212	OF--established patient, problem focused
82270	blood screening, occult; feces mod. -90		99213	OF--established patient, expanded
82947	glucose screening--quantitative		99214	OF--established patient, detailed...
82951	glucose tolerance test, three specimens		99215	OF--established patient, comprehensive..
83718	HDL cholesterol		99394	established patient, adolescent, per...
84478	triglycerides test		99396	established patient, 40-64 years, per...
85007	manual differential WBC			
85022	hemogram, automated, and manual...			

Payments $10 copay, check #456   **Remarks**

Diagnosis 531.30

ChampVA

No. 214778924

Date Oct. 4, 2004

Payable to: Family Care Center

$15.00

Fifteen and no/100 ———————————————————————— *dollars*

Stephenson Bank
Stephenson, OH 60089

Claim #07659A

021203347   0379 664 02   214778924

OhioCare HMO   *No.* 78901234
                                                   Date Oct. 4, 2004

Payable to: Family Care Center $2500.00

Two thousand five hundred and no/100 ——————————— *dollars*

Stephenson Bank
Stephenson, OH 60089

For 9/2004
021203347   0379 322 04   78901234

Blue Cross/Blue Shield
340 Boulevard
Columbus, OH 60220

Family Care Center
285 Stephenson Boulevard
Stephenson, OH 60089

Practice ID: 6078BFA

Date Prepared: 11/03/04

RA Number: 001234

Patient's Name	Dates of Service From - Thru	POS	Proc	Qty	Proc Charge	Amt Paid Provider
Giles, Sheila	10/29/04 - 10/29/04	11	99213	1	$72.00	$57.60
Giles, Sheila	10/29/04 - 10/29/04	11	71010	1	$91.00	$72.80
Giles, Sheila	10/29/04 - 10/29/04	11	86403	1	$58.00	$46.40
Simmons, Jill	10/29/04 - 10/29/04	11	99212	1	$54.00	$43.20
Simmons, Jill	10/29/04 - 10/29/04	11	87086	1	$51.00	$40.80

* * * * * * * *   *Check #8901 is attached in the amount of $260.80*   * * * * * * * *

East Ohio PPO
10 Central Avenue
Halevile, OH 60890

Family Care Center
285 Stephenson Boulevard
Stephenson, OH 60089

Practice ID: 01-234567

Date Prepared: 10/03/2004   **RA Number:** 101010

Patient's Name	Dates of Service From - Thru	POS	Proc	Qty	Proc Charge	Amt Paid Provider
Arlen, Susan	09/06/04 -09/06/04	11	99212	1	$46.00	$31.00
Bell, Herbert	09/06/04 -09/06/04	11	99211	1	$30.00	$15.00
Bell, Janine	09/06/04 -09/06/04	11	99213	1	$62.00	$47.00
Bell, Janine	09/06/04 -09/06/04	11	73510	1	$103.00	$103.00
Bell, Jonathan	09/06/04 -09/06/04	11	99394	1	$149.00	$134.00
Bell, Samuel	09/06/04 -09/06/04	11	99212	1	$46.00	$31.00
Bell, Sarina	09/06/04 -09/06/04	11	99213	1	$62.00	$47.00

* * * * * * *   *Check #4567890 is attached in the amount of $408.00*   * * * * * * *

Family Care Center
285 Stephenson Boulevard
Stephenson, OH 60089
(614)555-0000

Date: _11/12/2004_

Name _Anthony Battistuta_

Chart Number _BATTIANO_

Physician _Dr. McGrath_

01	patient payment, cash		85651	erythrocyte sedimentation rate--non-auto
02	patient payment, check		86403	strep test, quick
03	insurance carrier payment		86585	tuberculosis, tine test
04	insurance company adjustment		86588	direct streptococcus screen
05	adjustment, patient		87072	culture by commercial kit, nonurine...
12011	simple suture--face--local anes.		87076	bacterial culture, anerobic, with GC...
29125	application of short arm splint; static		(87086)	urine culture and colony count
29425	application of short leg cast, walking		90703	tetanus injection
45378	colonoscopy--diagnostic		90782	injection with material, subcutaneous or
45380	colonoscopy--with biopsy		92516	facial nerve function studies
50390	aspiration of renal cyst by needle		93000	Electrocardiogram--ECG with interpret...
71010	chest x-ray, single view, frontal		93015	Treadmill stress test, with physician...
71020	chest x-ray, two views, frontal & lat...		96900	ultraviolet light treatment
71030	chest x-ray, complete, four views		99070	supplies and materials provided
73070	elbow x-ray, AP and lateral views		99201	OF--new patient, problem focused
73090	forearm x-ray, AP and lateral views		99202	OF--new patient, expanded
73100	wrist x-ray, AP and lateral views		99203	OF--new patient, detailed history and...
73510	hip x-ray, complete, two views		99204	OF--new patient, comprehensive history..
73600	ankle x-ray, AP and lateral views		99205	OF--new patient, comprehensive history..
80019	19 clinical chemistry tests		99211	OF--established patient, minimal
80061	lipid panel		(99212)	OF--established patient, problem focused
82270	blood screening, occult; feces		99213	OF--established patient, expanded
82947	glucose screening--quantitative		99214	OF--established patient, detailed...
(82951)	glucose tolerance test, three specimens _mod. -90_		99215	OF--established patient, comprehensive..
83718	HDL cholesterol		99394	established patient, adolescent, per...
84478	triglycerides test		99396	established patient, 40-64 years, per...
85007	manual differential WBC			
85022	hemogram, automated, and manual...			

Payments _____

Remarks _New address:_
36 Grant Blvd.
Grandville, OH 60092
_(614) 029-3333_

Diagnosis _diabetes_

Family Care Center
285 Stephenson Boulevard
Stephenson, OH 60089
(614)555-0000

Date: 11/12/2004   **Name** Lawana Brooks

Chart Number BROOKLA0   **Physician** Dr. McGrath

01	patient payment, cash	85651	erythrocyte sedimentation rate--non-auto
02	patient payment, check	86403	strep test, quick
03	insurance carrier payment	86585	tuberculosis, tine test
04	insurance company adjustment	86588	direct streptococcus screen
05	adjustment, patient	87072	culture by commercial kit, nonurine...
12011	simple suture--face--local anes.	87076	bacterial culture, anerobic, with GC...
29125	application of short arm splint; static	87086	urine culture and colony count
29425	application of short leg cast, walking	90703	tetanus injection
45378	colonoscopy--diagnostic	90782	injection with material, subcutaneous or
45380	colonoscopy--with biopsy	92516	facial nerve function studies
50390	aspiration of renal cyst by needle	93000	Electrocardiogram--ECG with interpret...
71010	chest x-ray, single view, frontal	93015	Treadmill stress test, with physician...
71020	chest x-ray, two views, frontal & lat...	96900	ultraviolet light treatment
71030	chest x-ray, complete, four views	99070	supplies and materials provided
73070	elbow x-ray, AP and lateral views	99201	OF--new patient, problem focused
73090	forearm x-ray, AP and lateral views	99202	OF--new patient, expanded
73100	wrist x-ray, AP and lateral views	99203	OF--new patient, detailed history and...
73510	hip x-ray, complete, two views	99204	OF--new patient, comprehensive history..
73600	ankle x-ray, AP and lateral views	99205	OF--new patient, comprehensive history..
80019	19 clinical chemistry tests	99211	OF--established patient, minimal
80061	lipid panel	99212	OF--established patient, problem focused
82270	blood screening, occult; feces	99213	OF--established patient, expanded
82947	glucose screening--quantitative	99214	OF--established patient, detailed...
82951	glucose tolerance test, three specimens	99215	OF--established patient, comprehensive..
83718	HDL cholesterol	99394	established patient, adolescent, per...
84478	triglycerides test	99396	established patient, 40-64 years, per...
85007	manual differential WBC		
85022	hemogram, automated, and manual...		

Payments _____   **Remarks** See case notes

Diagnosis 841.0 / E885 / E849.3

SOURCE DOCUMENT 12

Lawana Brooks - Case Notes

Date: 11/12/2004
Description: Fall at work - WC
Date of Injury: 11/12/2004
Nature of Injury: Work Injury/Non-collision
Nature of Visit: Emergency

Family Care Center
285 Stephenson Boulevard
Stephenson, OH 60089
(614)555-0000

Date: 11/12/2004   Name: Edwin Hsu

Chart Number: HSUEDWIO   Physician: Dr. McGrath

01	patient payment, cash		85651	erythrocyte sedimentation rate--non-auto
02	patient payment, check		86403	strep test, quick
03	insurance carrier payment		86585	tuberculosis, tine test
04	insurance company adjustment		86588	direct streptococcus screen
05	adjustment, patient		87072	culture by commercial kit, nonurine...
12011	simple suture--face--local anes.		87076	bacterial culture, anerobic, with GC...
29125	application of short arm splint; static		87086	urine culture and colony count
29425	application of short leg cast, walking		90703	tetanus injection
45378	colonoscopy--diagnostic		90782	injection with material, subcutaneous or
45380	colonoscopy--with biopsy		92516	facial nerve function studies
50390	aspiration of renal cyst by needle		93000	Electrocardiogram--ECG with interpret...
71010	chest x-ray, single view, frontal		93015	Treadmill stress test, with physician...
71020	chest x-ray, two views, frontal & lat...		96900	ultraviolet light treatment
71030	chest x-ray, complete, four views		99070	supplies and materials provided
73070	elbow x-ray, AP and lateral views		99201	OF--new patient, problem focused
73090	forearm x-ray, AP and lateral views		99202	OF--new patient, expanded
73100	wrist x-ray, AP and lateral views		99203	OF--new patient, detailed history and...
73510	hip x-ray, complete, two views		99204	OF--new patient, comprehensive history..
73600	ankle x-ray, AP and lateral views		99205	OF--new patient, comprehensive history..
80019	19 clinical chemistry tests		99211	OF--established patient, minimal
80061	lipid panel		99212	OF--established patient, problem focused
82270	blood screening, occult; feces		99213	OF--established patient, expanded
82947	glucose screening--quantitative		99214	OF--established patient, detailed...
82951	glucose tolerance test, three specimens		99215	OF--established patient, comprehensive..
83718	HDL cholesterol		99394	established patient, adolescent, per...
84478	triglycerides test		99396	established patient, 40-64 years, per...
85007	manual differential WBC			
85022	hemogram, automated, and manual...			

Payments: $20 copay, check #1066   Remarks: see case notes

Diagnosis: 461.9, acute sinusitis

SOURCE DOCUMENT 14

Edwin Hsu - Case Notes

Date: 11/12/2004
Description: Acute sinusitis

Change Patient's Address

New Address: 56 Reynolds St.
                      Stephenson, OH 60089
                      614-034-6729

Add New Insurance Carrier to Database

Code: 16
Name: Midwest Select
Address: 1245 Mohawk Lane
                      Columbus, OH 60625
Phone: 614-555-1211
Practice ID: 12345678

Plan Name: Midwest Select HMO
Type: HMO
Procedure Code Set: 1
Diagnosis Code Set: 1
Signature on File: Signature on file
Default Billing Method: Electronic
Print PINS on Forms: Provider Name and PIN

EMC Receiver: 0000 - National Data Corporation
EMC Payor Number: 50678
EMC Sub ID: 5034
NDC Record Code: 01
Payment: 03 - insurance carrier payment
Adjustment: MIDADJ - Midwest Select Adjustment

McGrath PIN/Group ID 1234 / 5560
Beach PIN/Group ID   5678 / 5560
Banu PIN/Group ID   9012 / 5560

Create New Case

Price Code: A

Policy Number   51249
Group Number   256
Policy Dates, Start   11/12/2004
Accept Assignment: Yes
Capitated Plan: Yes
Copayment Amount: 20.00
Insurance Coverage by 80%
  Service Classification

PATIENT INFORMATION FORM

THIS SECTION REFERS TO PATIENT ONLY

Name: Hannah Syzmanski	Sex: F	Marital status: ☒ S ☐ M ☐ D ☐ W	Birth date: 2/26/88

Address: 3 Broadbrook Lane	SS#: 907-66-0003

City: Stephenson	State: OH	Zip: 60089	Employer:

Home phone: 614-086-4444	Employer's address:

614-555-1001	City:	State:	Zip:

Spouse's name:	Spouse's employer:

Emergency contact:	Relationship:	Phone #:

FILL IN IF PATIENT IS A MINOR

Parent/Guardian's name: Michael Syzmanski	Sex: M	Marital status: ☐ S ☒ M ☐ D ☐ W	Birth date: 6/5/72

Phone: 614-086-4444	SS#: 022-45-6789

Address: 3 Broadbrook Lane	

City: Stephenson	State: OH	Zip: 60089	Employer Nichol's Hardware

Student status: Full-time	City: Stephenson	State: OH	Zip: 60089

INSURANCE INFORMATION

Primary insurance company:	Secondary insurance company:

Policyholder's name:	Birth date:	Policyholder's name:	Birth date:

Copayment:	Price Code:	Copayment:	Price Code:

Policy #:	Group #:	Policy #:	Group #:

OTHER INFORMATION

Reason for visit: Physical	Allergy to medication (list): bee stings

Name of referring physician: Dr. Harold Gearhart	If auto accident, list date and state in which it occurred:

Michael Syzmanski
_____
(Patient's signature/Parent or guardian's signature)

11/12/2004
_____
(Date)

Family Care Center
285 Stephenson Boulevard
Stephenson, OH 60089
(614)555-0000

Date: 11/12/2004

Name Hannah Syzmanski

Chart Number SYZMAHAO

Physician Dr. Banu

01	patient payment, cash	85651	erythrocyte sedimentation rate--non-auto
02	patient payment, check	86403	strep test, quick
03	insurance carrier payment	86585	tuberculosis, tine test
04	insurance company adjustment	86588	direct streptococcus screen
05	adjustment, patient	87072	culture by commercial kit, nonurine...
12011	simple suture--face--local anes.	87076	bacterial culture, anerobic, with GC...
29125	application of short arm splint; static	87086	urine culture and colony count
29425	application of short leg cast, walking	90703	tetanus injection
45378	colonoscopy--diagnostic	90782	injection with material, subcutaneous or
45380	colonoscopy--with biopsy	92516	facial nerve function studies
50390	aspiration of renal cyst by needle	93000	Electrocardiogram--ECG with interpret...
71010	chest x-ray, single view, frontal	93015	Treadmill stress test, with physician...
71020	chest x-ray, two views, frontal & lat...	96900	ultraviolet light treatment
71030	chest x-ray, complete, four views	99070	supplies and materials provided
73070	elbow x-ray, AP and lateral views	99201	OF--new patient, problem focused
73090	forearm x-ray, AP and lateral views	99202	OF--new patient, expanded
73100	wrist x-ray, AP and lateral views	99203	OF--new patient, detailed history and...
73510	hip x-ray, complete, two views	99204	OF--new patient, comprehensive history..
73600	ankle x-ray, AP and lateral views	99205	OF--new patient, comprehensive history..
80019	19 clinical chemistry tests	99211	OF--established patient, minimal
80061	lipid panel	99212	OF--established patient, problem focused
82270	blood screening, occult; feces	99213	OF--established patient, expanded
82947	glucose screening--quantitative	99214	OF--established patient, detailed...
82951	glucose tolerance test, three specimens	99215	OF--established patient, comprehensive..
83718	HDL cholesterol	99394	established patient, adolescent, per...
84478	triglycerides test	99396	established patient, 40-64 years, per...
85007	manual differential WBC		
85022	hemogram, automated, and manual...		

Payments $15 copay, check #3019

Remarks

Diagnosis v70.0

Family Care Center
285 Stephenson Boulevard
Stephenson, OH 60089
(614)555-0000

Date: 11/15/2004

Name Carlos Lopez

Chart Number LOPEZCAO

Physician Dr. McGrath

Code	Description	Code	Description
01	patient payment, cash	85651	erythrocyte sedimentation rate--non-auto
02	patient payment, check	86403	strep test, quick
03	insurance carrier payment	86585	tuberculosis, tine test
04	insurance company adjustment	86588	direct streptococcus screen
05	adjustment, patient	87072	culture by commercial kit, nonurine...
12011	simple suture--face--local anes.	87076	bacterial culture, anaerobic, with GC...
29125	application of short arm splint; static	87086	urine culture and colony count
29425	application of short leg cast, walking	90703	tetanus injection
45378	colonoscopy--diagnostic	90782	injection with material, subcutaneous or
45380	colonoscopy--with biopsy	92516	facial nerve function studies
50390	aspiration of renal cyst by needle	(93000)	Electrocardiogram--ECG with interpret...
71010	chest x-ray, single view, frontal	93015	Treadmill stress test, with physician...
71020	chest x-ray, two views, frontal & lat...	96900	ultraviolet light treatment
71030	chest x-ray, complete, four views	99070	supplies and materials provided
73070	elbow x-ray, AP and lateral views	99201	OF--new patient, problem focused
73090	forearm x-ray, AP and lateral views	99202	OF--new patient, expanded
73100	wrist x-ray, AP and lateral views	99203	OF--new patient, detailed history and...
73510	hip x-ray, complete, two views	99204	OF--new patient, comprehensive history..
73600	ankle x-ray, AP and lateral views	99205	OF--new patient, comprehensive history..
80019	19 clinical chemistry tests	99211	OF--established patient, minimal
80061	lipid panel	(99212)	OF--established patient, problem focused
82270	blood screening, occult; feces	99213	OF--established patient, expanded
82947	glucose screening--quantitative	99214	OF--established patient, detailed...
82951	glucose tolerance test, three specimens	99215	OF--established patient, comprehensive..
83718	HDL cholesterol	99394	established patient, adolescent, per...
84478	triglycerides test	99396	established patient, 40-64 years, per...
85007	manual differential WBC		
85022	hemogram, automated, and manual...		

Payments $15 copay, check #1001

Remarks Patient had palpitations

Diagnosis v65.5, patient fears unfounded

PATIENT INFORMATION FORM

THIS SECTION REFERS TO PATIENT ONLY

Name: Christopher Palmer			Sex: M	Marital status: ☒ S ☐ M ☐ D ☐ W	Birth date: 1/5/48
Address: 17 Red Oak Lane			SS#: 607-49-7620		
City: Jefferson	State: OH	Zip: 60093	Employer: unemployed - disabled		
Home phone: 614-077-2249			Employer's address:		
			City:	State:	Zip:
Spouse's name:			Spouse's employer:		
Emergency contact:			Relationship:		Phone #:

FILL IN IF PATIENT IS A MINOR

Parent/Guardian's name:			Sex:	Marital status: ☐ S ☐ M ☐ D ☐ W	Birth date:
Phone:			SS#:		
Address:					
City:	State:	Zip:	Employer		
Student status:			City:	State:	Zip:

INSURANCE INFORMATION

Primary insurance company: Medicaid		Secondary insurance company:	
Policyholder's name: Christopher Palmer	Birth date: 1/5/48	Policyholder's name:	Birth date:
Copayment:	Price Code: D	Copayment:	Price Code:
Policy #: 607497620	Group #:	Policy #:	Group #:

OTHER INFORMATION

Reason for visit: Trouble breathing	Allergy to medication (list):
Name of referring physician: Dr. Marion Davis	If auto accident, list date and state in which it occurred:

Christopher Palmer

(Patient's signature/Parent or guardian's signature)

_11/12/2004_

(Date)

Family Care Center
285 Stephenson Boulevard
Stephenson, OH 60089
(614)555-0000

Date: 11/12/2004

Name Christopher Palmer

Chart Number PALMECHO

Physician Dr. Beach

01	patient payment, cash	85651	erythrocyte sedimentation rate--non-auto
02	patient payment, check	86403	strep test, quick
03	insurance carrier payment	86585	tuberculosis, tine test
04	insurance company adjustment	86588	direct streptococcus screen
05	adjustment, patient	87072	culture by commercial kit, nonurine...
12011	simple suture--face--local anes.	87076	bacterial culture, anerobic, with GC...
29125	application of short arm splint; static	87086	urine culture and colony count
29425	application of short leg cast, walking	90703	tetanus injection
45378	colonoscopy--diagnostic	90782	injection with material, subcutaneous or
45380	colonoscopy--with biopsy	92516	facial nerve function studies
50390	aspiration of renal cyst by needle	93000	Electrocardiogram--ECG with interpret...
71010	chest x-ray, single view, frontal	93015	Treadmill stress test, with physician...
71020	chest x-ray, two views, frontal & lat...	96900	ultraviolet light treatment
71030	chest x-ray, complete, four views	99070	supplies and materials provided
73070	elbow x-ray, AP and lateral views	99201	OF--new patient, problem focused
73090	forearm x-ray, AP and lateral views	99202	OF--new patient, expanded
73100	wrist x-ray, AP and lateral views	99203	OF--new patient, detailed history and...
73510	hip x-ray, complete, two views	99204	OF--new patient, comprehensive history..
73600	ankle x-ray, AP and lateral views	99205	OF--new patient, comprehensive history..
80019	19 clinical chemistry tests	99211	OF--established patient, minimal
80061	lipid panel	99212	OF--established patient, problem focused
82270	blood screening, occult; feces	99213	OF--established patient, expanded
82947	glucose screening--quantitative	99214	OF--established patient, detailed...
82951	glucose tolerance test, three specimens	99215	OF--established patient, comprehensive..
83718	HDL cholesterol	99394	established patient, adolescent, per...
84478	triglycerides test	99396	established patient, 40-64 years, per...
85007	manual differential WBC		
85022	hemogram, automated, and manual...		

Payments _____

Remarks _____

Diagnosis 485, bronchopneumonia

East Ohio PPO
10 Central Avenue
Halevile, OH 60890

Family Care Center
285 Stephenson Boulevard
Stephenson, OH 60089

Practice ID: 01-234567

Date Prepared: 11/11/2004   **RA Number:** 102010

Patient's Name	Dates of Service From - Thru	POS	Proc	Qty	Proc Charge	Amt Paid Provider
Brooks, Lawana	10/29/04 -10/29/04	11	73600	1	$80.00	$64.00
Brooks, Lawana	10/29/04 -10/29/04	11	99212	1	$46.00	$36.80
Hsu, Diane	10/29/04 -10/29/04	11	80019	1	$80.00	$64.00
Hsu, Diane	10/29/04 -10/29/04	11	99213	1	$62.00	$49.60
Syzmanski, Michael	10/29/04 -10/29/04	11	99212	1	$46.00	$36.80

* * * * * * * *   *Check #4679323 is attached in the amount of $251.20*   * * * * * * * *

Family Care Center
285 Stephenson Boulevard
Stephenson, OH 60089
(614)555-0000

Date: 11/15/2004   **Name** Diane Hsu

Chart Number HSUDIANO   **Physician** Dr. McGrath

01	patient payment, cash		85651	erythrocyte sedimentation rate--non-auto
02	patient payment, check		86403	strep test, quick
03	insurance carrier payment		86585	tuberculosis, tine test
04	insurance company adjustment		86588	direct streptococcus screen
05	adjustment, patient		(87072)	culture by commercial kit, nonurine...
12011	simple suture--face--local anes.		87076	bacterial culture, anaerobic, with GC...
29125	application of short arm splint; static		87086	urine culture and colony count
29425	application of short leg cast, walking		90703	tetanus injection
45378	colonoscopy--diagnostic		90782	injection with material, subcutaneous or
45380	colonoscopy--with biopsy		92516	facial nerve function studies
50390	aspiration of renal cyst by needle		93000	Electrocardiogram--ECG with interpret...
71010	chest x-ray, single view, frontal		93015	Treadmill stress test, with physician...
71020	chest x-ray, two views, frontal & lat...		96900	ultraviolet light treatment
71030	chest x-ray, complete, four views		99070	supplies and materials provided
73070	elbow x-ray, AP and lateral views		99201	OF--new patient, problem focused
73090	forearm x-ray, AP and lateral views		99202	OF--new patient, expanded
73100	wrist x-ray, AP and lateral views		99203	OF--new patient, detailed history and...
73510	hip x-ray, complete, two views		99204	OF--new patient, comprehensive history..
73600	ankle x-ray, AP and lateral views		99205	OF--new patient, comprehensive history..
80019	19 clinical chemistry tests		99211	OF--established patient, minimal
80061	lipid panel		(99212)	OF--established patient, problem focused
82270	blood screening, occult; feces		99213	OF--established patient, expanded
82947	glucose screening--quantitative		99214	OF--established patient, detailed...
82951	glucose tolerance test, three specimens		99215	OF--established patient, comprehensive..
83718	HDL cholesterol		99394	established patient, adolescent, per...
84478	triglycerides test		99396	established patient, 40-64 years, per...
85007	manual differential WBC			
85022	hemogram, automated, and manual...			

Payments $20 copay, check #3419   **Remarks** Next appt. 1 week from today, 2:00 p.m., 15 minutes

Diagnosis 487.1, influenza

Family Care Center
285 Stephenson Boulevard
Stephenson, OH 60089
(614)555-0000

Date: 11/15/2004

Chart Number SYZMAMIO

Name Michael Syzmanski

Physician Dr. Banu

01	patient payment, cash	85651	erythrocyte sedimentation rate--non-auto
02	patient payment, check	86403	strep test, quick
03	insurance carrier payment	86585	tuberculosis, tine test
04	insurance company adjustment	86588	direct streptococcus screen
05	adjustment, patient	87072	culture by commercial kit, nonurine...
12011	simple suture--face--local anes.	87076	bacterial culture, anaerobic, with GC...
29125	application of short arm splint; static	87086	urine culture and colony count
29425	application of short leg cast, walking	90703	tetanus injection
45378	colonoscopy--diagnostic	90782	injection with material, subcutaneous or
45380	colonoscopy--with biopsy	92516	facial nerve function studies
50390	aspiration of renal cyst by needle	93000	Electrocardiogram--ECG with interpret...
71010	chest x-ray, single view, frontal	93015	Treadmill stress test, with physician...
71020	chest x-ray, two views, frontal & lat...	96900	ultraviolet light treatment
71030	chest x-ray, complete, four views	99070	supplies and materials provided
73070	elbow x-ray, AP and lateral views	99201	OF--new patient, problem focused
73090	forearm x-ray, AP and lateral views	99202	OF--new patient, expanded
73100	wrist x-ray, AP and lateral views	99203	OF--new patient, detailed history and...
73510	hip x-ray, complete, two views	99204	OF--new patient, comprehensive history..
73600	ankle x-ray, AP and lateral views	99205	OF--new patient, comprehensive history..
80019	19 clinical chemistry tests	99211	OF--established patient, minimal
80061	lipid panel	99212	OF--established patient, problem focused
82270	blood screening, occult; feces	99213	OF--established patient, expanded
82947	glucose screening--quantitative	99214	OF--established patient, detailed...
82951	glucose tolerance test, three specimens	99215	OF--established patient, comprehensive..
83718	HDL cholesterol	99394	established patient, adolescent, per...
84478	triglycerides test	99396	established patient, 40-64 years, per...
85007	manual differential WBC		
85022	hemogram, automated, and manual...		

Payments $15 copay, check #3119

Diagnosis 455.6, hemorrhoids

Remarks rectal bleeding, first experienced 11/10/2004

PATIENT INFORMATION FORM

THIS SECTION REFERS TO PATIENT ONLY

Name: Stewart Robertson	Sex: M	Marital status: ☐ S ☐ M ☒ D ☐ W	Birth date: 12/21/63

Address: 109 West Central Ave.	SS#: 920-39-4567

City: Stephenson	State: OH	Zip: 60089	Employer: Nichols Hardware

Home phone: 614-022-3111	Employer's address:
	City:	State:	Zip:

Spouse's name:	Spouse's employer:

Emergency contact:	Relationship:	Phone #:

FILL IN IF PATIENT IS A MINOR

Parent/Guardian's name:	Sex:	Marital status: ☐ S ☐ M ☐ D ☐ W	Birth date:

Phone:	SS#:

Address:	

City:	State:	Zip:	Employer

Student status:	City:	State:	Zip:

INSURANCE INFORMATION

Primary insurance company: OhioCare HMO	Secondary insurance company:

Policyholder's name: Stewart Robertson	Birth date: 12/21/63	Policyholder's name:	Birth date:

Copayment: $15	Price Code: A	Copayment:	Price Code:

Policy #: 607497620	Group #:	Policy #:	Group #:

OTHER INFORMATION

Reason for visit: Routine physical	Allergy to medication (list):

Name of referring physician: Dr. Janet Wood	If auto accident, list date and state in which it occurred:

Stewart Robertson   12/10/04

(Patient's signature/Parent or guardian's signature)   (Date)

Family Care Center
285 Stephenson Boulevard
Stephenson, OH 60089
(614)555-0000

Date: 12/18/04

Name Stewart Robertson

Chart Number ROBERSTO

Physician Dr. Beach

01	patient payment, cash		85651	erythrocyte sedimentation rate--non-auto
02	patient payment, check		86403	strep test, quick
03	insurance carrier payment		86585	tuberculosis, tine test
04	insurance company adjustment		86588	direct streptococcus screen
05	adjustment, patient		87072	culture by commercial kit, nonurine...
12011	simple suture--face--local anes.		87076	bacterial culture, anerobic, with GC...
29125	application of short arm splint; static		87086	urine culture and colony count
29425	application of short leg cast, walking		90703	tetanus injection
45378	colonoscopy--diagnostic		90782	injection with material, subcutaneous or
45380	colonoscopy--with biopsy		92516	facial nerve function studies
50390	aspiration of renal cyst by needle		(93000)	Electrocardiogram--ECG with interpret...
71010	chest x-ray, single view, frontal		93015	Treadmill stress test, with physician...
71020	chest x-ray, two views, frontal & lat...		96900	ultraviolet light treatment
71030	chest x-ray, complete, four views		99070	supplies and materials provided
73070	elbow x-ray, AP and lateral views		99201	OF--new patient, problem focused
73090	forearm x-ray, AP and lateral views		99202	OF--new patient, expanded
73100	wrist x-ray, AP and lateral views		(99203)	OF--new patient, detailed history and...
73510	hip x-ray, complete, two views		99204	OF--new patient, comprehensive history..
73600	ankle x-ray, AP and lateral views		99205	OF--new patient, comprehensive history..
80019	19 clinical chemistry tests		99211	OF--established patient, minimal
80061	lipid panel		99212	OF--established patient, problem focused
82270	blood screening, occult; feces		99213	OF--established patient, expanded
82947	glucose screening--quantitative		99214	OF--established patient, detailed...
82951	glucose tolerance test, three specimens		99215	OF--established patient, comprehensive..
83718	HDL cholesterol		99394	established patient, adolescent, per...
84478	triglycerides test		99396	established patient, 40-64 years, per...
85007	manual differential WBC			
85022	hemogram, automated, and manual...			

Payments $15 copay, check #416

Remarks

Diagnosis v70.0

Family Care Center
285 Stephenson Boulevard
Stephenson, OH 60089
(614)555-0000

Date: 12/18/04   **Name** Michael Syzmanski

Chart Number SYZMAMIO   **Physician** Dr. McGrath

01	patient payment, cash	85651	erythrocyte sedimentation rate--non-auto
02	patient payment, check	86403	strep test, quick
03	insurance carrier payment	86585	tuberculosis, tine test
04	insurance company adjustment	86588	direct streptococcus screen
05	adjustment, patient	87072	culture by commercial kit, nonurine...
12011	simple suture--face--local anes.	87076	bacterial culture, anerobic, with GC...
29125	application of short arm splint; static	87086	urine culture and colony count
29425	application of short leg cast, walking	90703	tetanus injection
45378	colonoscopy--diagnostic	90782	injection with material, subcutaneous or
45380	colonoscopy--with biopsy	92516	facial nerve function studies
50390	aspiration of renal cyst by needle	93000	Electrocardiogram--ECG with interpret...
71010	chest x-ray, single view, frontal	93015	Treadmill stress test, with physician...
71020	chest x-ray, two views, frontal & lat...	96900	ultraviolet light treatment
71030	chest x-ray, complete, four views	99070	supplies and materials provided
73070	elbow x-ray, AP and lateral views	99201	OF--new patient, problem focused
73090	forearm x-ray, AP and lateral views	99202	OF--new patient, expanded
73100	wrist x-ray, AP and lateral views	99203	OF--new patient, detailed history and...
73510	hip x-ray, complete, two views	99204	OF--new patient, comprehensive history..
73600	ankle x-ray, AP and lateral views	99205	OF--new patient, comprehensive history..
80019	19 clinical chemistry tests	99211	OF--established patient, minimal
80061	lipid panel	99212	OF--established patient, problem focused
82270	blood screening, occult; feces	99213	OF--established patient, expanded
82947	glucose screening--quantitative	99214	OF--established patient, detailed...
82951	glucose tolerance test, three specimens	99215	OF--established patient, comprehensive..
83718	HDL cholesterol	99394	established patient, adolescent, per...
84478	triglycerides test	99396	established patient, 40-64 years, per...
85007	manual differential WBC		
85022	hemogram, automated, and manual...		

Payments $15 copay, check #3139   **Remarks**

Diagnosis 870.8

Family Care Center
285 Stephenson Boulevard
Stephenson, OH 60089
(614)555-0000

Date: 1/05/05

Name Luther Jackson

Chart Number JACKSLU0

Physician Dr. Banu

01	patient payment, cash		85651	erythrocyte sedimentation rate--non-auto
02	patient payment, check		86403	strep test, quick
03	insurance carrier payment		86585	tuberculosis, tine test
04	insurance company adjustment		86588	direct streptococcus screen
05	adjustment, patient		87072	culture by commercial kit, nonurine...
12011	simple suture--face--local anes.		87076	bacterial culture, anerobic, with GC...
29125	application of short arm splint; static		87086	urine culture and colony count
29425	application of short leg cast, walking		90703	tetanus injection
45378	colonoscopy--diagnostic		90782	injection with material, subcutaneous or
45380	colonoscopy--with biopsy		92516	facial nerve function studies
50390	aspiration of renal cyst by needle		93000	Electrocardiogram--ECG with interpret...
71010	chest x-ray, single view, frontal		93015	Treadmill stress test, with physician...
(71020)	chest x-ray, two views, frontal & lat...		96900	ultraviolet light treatment
71030	chest x-ray, complete, four views		99070	supplies and materials provided
73070	elbow x-ray, AP and lateral views		99201	OF--new patient, problem focused
73090	forearm x-ray, AP and lateral views		99202	OF--new patient, expanded
73100	wrist x-ray, AP and lateral views		99203	OF--new patient, detailed history and...
73510	hip x-ray, complete, two views		99204	OF--new patient, comprehensive history..
73600	ankle x-ray, AP and lateral views		99205	OF--new patient, comprehensive history..
80019	19 clinical chemistry tests		99211	OF--established patient, minimal
80061	lipid panel		(99212)	OF--established patient, problem focused
82270	blood screening, occult; feces		99213	OF--established patient, expanded
82947	glucose screening--quantitative		99214	OF--established patient, detailed...
82951	glucose tolerance test, three specimens		99215	OF--established patient, comprehensive..
83718	HDL cholesterol		99394	established patient, adolescent, per...
84478	triglycerides test		99396	established patient, 40-64 years, per...
85007	manual differential WBC			
85022	hemogram, automated, and manual...			

Payments $15 copay, check #1291

Remarks

Diagnosis 485, bronchopneumonia

Family Care Center
285 Stephenson Boulevard
Stephenson, OH 60089
(614)555-0000

Date: 1/5/05   **Name** Jill Simmons

Chart Number SIMMOJIO   **Physician** Dr. Beach

01	patient payment, cash		85651	erythrocyte sedimentation rate--non-auto
02	patient payment, check		86403	strep test, quick
03	insurance carrier payment		86585	tuberculosis, tine test
04	insurance company adjustment		86588	direct streptococcus screen
05	adjustment, patient		87072	culture by commercial kit, nonurine...
12011	simple suture--face--local anes.		87076	bacterial culture, anaerobic, with GC...
29125	application of short arm splint; static		87086	urine culture and colony count
29425	application of short leg cast, walking		90703	tetanus injection
45378	colonoscopy--diagnostic		90782	injection with material, subcutaneous or
45380	colonoscopy--with biopsy		92516	facial nerve function studies
50390	aspiration of renal cyst by needle		93000	Electrocardiogram--ECG with interpret...
71010	chest x-ray, single view, frontal		93015	Treadmill stress test, with physician...
71020	chest x-ray, two views, frontal & lat...		96900	ultraviolet light treatment
71030	chest x-ray, complete, four views		99070	supplies and materials provided
73070	elbow x-ray, AP and lateral views		99201	OF--new patient, problem focused
73090	forearm x-ray, AP and lateral views		99202	OF--new patient, expanded
73100	wrist x-ray, AP and lateral views		99203	OF--new patient, detailed history and...
73510	hip x-ray, complete, two views		99204	OF--new patient, comprehensive history..
73600	ankle x-ray, AP and lateral views		99205	OF--new patient, comprehensive history..
80019	19 clinical chemistry tests		99211	OF--established patient, minimal
80061	lipid panel		99212	OF--established patient, problem focused
82270	blood screening, occult; feces		99213	OF--established patient, expanded
82947	glucose screening--quantitative		99214	OF--established patient, detailed...
82951	glucose tolerance test, three specimens		99215	OF--established patient, comprehensive..
83718	HDL cholesterol		99394	established patient, adolescent, per...
84478	triglycerides test		99396	established patient, 40-64 years, per...
85007	manual differential WBC			
85022	hemogram, automated, and manual...			

Payments _____   **Remarks** _____

Diagnosis 034.0, strep sore throat

Family Care Center
285 Stephenson Boulevard
Stephenson, OH 60089
(614)555-0000

Date: 1/5/05

Name Nancy Stern

Chart Number STERNNA0

Physician Dr. McGrath

01	patient payment, cash		85651	erythrocyte sedimentation rate--non-auto
02	patient payment, check		86403	strep test, quick
03	insurance carrier payment		86585	tuberculosis, tine test
04	insurance company adjustment		86588	direct streptococcus screen
05	adjustment, patient		87072	culture by commercial kit, nonurine...
12011	simple suture--face--local anes.		87076	bacterial culture, anerobic, with GC...
29125	application of short arm splint; static		(87086)	urine culture and colony count
29425	application of short leg cast, walking		90703	tetanus injection
45378	colonoscopy--diagnostic		90782	injection with material, subcutaneous or
45380	colonoscopy--with biopsy		92516	facial nerve function studies
50390	aspiration of renal cyst by needle		(93000)	Electrocardiogram--ECG with interpret...
71010	chest x-ray, single view, frontal		93015	Treadmill stress test, with physician...
71020	chest x-ray, two views, frontal & lat...		96900	ultraviolet light treatment
71030	chest x-ray, complete, four views		99070	supplies and materials provided
73070	elbow x-ray, AP and lateral views		99201	OF--new patient, problem focused
73090	forearm x-ray, AP and lateral views		99202	OF--new patient, expanded
73100	wrist x-ray, AP and lateral views		99203	OF--new patient, detailed history and...
73510	hip x-ray, complete, two views		99204	OF--new patient, comprehensive history..
73600	ankle x-ray, AP and lateral views		99205	OF--new patient, comprehensive history..
80019	19 clinical chemistry tests		99211	OF--established patient, minimal
80061	lipid panel		(99212)	OF--established patient, problem focused
82270	blood screening, occult; feces		99213	OF--established patient, expanded
82947	glucose screening--quantitative		99214	OF--established patient, detailed...
82951	glucose tolerance test, three specimens		99215	OF--established patient, comprehensive..
(83718	HDL cholesterol) mod. -90		99394	established patient, adolescent, per...
84478	triglycerides test		99396	established patient, 40-64 years, per...
(85007	manual differential WBC) mod. -90			
85022	hemogram, automated, and manual...			

Payments $15 copay, check #1022

Remarks

Diagnosis v70.0

Family Care Center
285 Stephenson Boulevard
Stephenson, OH 60089
(614)555-0000

Date: 1/5/05

Name Deborah Syzmanski

Chart Number SYZMADEO

Physician Dr. Banu

01	patient payment, cash		85651	erythrocyte sedimentation rate--non-auto
02	patient payment, check		86403	strep test, quick
03	insurance carrier payment		86585	tuberculosis, tine test
04	insurance company adjustment		86588	direct streptococcus screen
05	adjustment, patient		87072	culture by commercial kit, nonurine...
12011	simple suture--face--local anes.		87076	bacterial culture, anerobic, with GC...
29125	application of short arm splint; static		87086	urine culture and colony count
29425	application of short leg cast, walking		90703	tetanus injection
45378	colonoscopy--diagnostic		90782	injection with material, subcutaneous or
45380	colonoscopy--with biopsy		92516	facial nerve function studies
50390	aspiration of renal cyst by needle		93000	Electrocardiogram--ECG with interpret...
71010	chest x-ray, single view, frontal		93015	Treadmill stress test, with physician...
71020	chest x-ray, two views, frontal & lat...		96900	ultraviolet light treatment
71030	chest x-ray, complete, four views		99070	supplies and materials provided
73070	elbow x-ray, AP and lateral views		99201	OF--new patient, problem focused
73090	forearm x-ray, AP and lateral views		99202	OF--new patient, expanded
73100	wrist x-ray, AP and lateral views		99203	OF--new patient, detailed history and...
73510	hip x-ray, complete, two views		99204	OF--new patient, comprehensive history..
73600	ankle x-ray, AP and lateral views		99205	OF--new patient, comprehensive history..
80019	19 clinical chemistry tests		99211	OF--established patient, minimal
80061	lipid panel		99212	OF--established patient, problem focused
82270	blood screening, occult; feces		99213	OF--established patient, expanded
82947	glucose screening--quantitative		99214	OF--established patient, detailed...
82951	glucose tolerance test, three specimens		99215	OF--established patient, comprehensive..
83718	HDL cholesterol		99394	established patient, adolescent, per...
84478	triglycerides test		99396	established patient, 40-64 years, per...
85007	manual differential WBC			
85022	hemogram, automated, and manual,..			

Payments $15 copay, check #3219

Remarks

Diagnosis v70.0

Family Care Center
285 Stephenson Boulevard
Stephenson, OH 60089
(614)555-0000

Date: 1/5/05

Name Sheila Giles

Chart Number GILESSHO

Physician Dr. Beach

01	patient payment, cash	85651	erythrocyte sedimentation rate--non-auto
02	patient payment, check	86403	strep test, quick
03	insurance carrier payment	86585	tuberculosis, tine test
04	insurance company adjustment	86588	direct streptococcus screen
05	adjustment, patient	87072	culture by commercial kit, nonurine...
12011	simple suture--face--local anes.	87076	bacterial culture, anerobic, with GC...
29125	application of short arm splint; static	87086	urine culture and colony count
29425	application of short leg cast, walking	90703	tetanus injection
45378	colonoscopy--diagnostic	90782	injection with material, subcutaneous or
45380	colonoscopy--with biopsy	92516	facial nerve function studies
50390	aspiration of renal cyst by needle	93000	Electrocardiogram--ECG with interpret...
71010	chest x-ray, single view, frontal	93015	Treadmill stress test, with physician...
71020	chest x-ray, two views, frontal & lat...	96900	ultraviolet light treatment
71030	chest x-ray, complete, four views	99070	supplies and materials provided
73070	elbow x-ray, AP and lateral views	99201	OF--new patient, problem focused
73090	forearm x-ray, AP and lateral views	99202	OF--new patient, expanded
73100	wrist x-ray, AP and lateral views	99203	OF--new patient, detailed history and...
73510	hip x-ray, complete, two views	99204	OF--new patient, comprehensive history..
73600	ankle x-ray, AP and lateral views	99205	OF--new patient, comprehensive history..
80019	19 clinical chemistry tests	99211	OF--established patient, minimal
80061	lipid panel	99212	OF--established patient, problem focused
82270	blood screening, occult; feces	99213	OF--established patient, expanded
82947	glucose screening--quantitative	99214	OF--established patient, detailed...
82951	glucose tolerance test, three specimens	99215	OF--established patient, comprehensive..
83718	HDL cholesterol	99394	established patient, adolescent, per...
84478	triglycerides test	99396	established patient, 40-64 years, per...
85007	manual differential WBC		
85022	hemogram, automated, and manual...		

Payments _____

Remarks _____

Diagnosis V03.7

_____

Family Care Center
285 Stephenson Boulevard
Stephenson, OH 60089
(614)555-0000

Date: 1/5/05

Name Pauline Battistuta

Chart Number BATTIPAO

Physician Dr. McGrath

01	patient payment, cash	85651	erythrocyte sedimentation rate--non-auto
02	patient payment, check	86403	strep test, quick
03	insurance carrier payment	86585	tuberculosis, tine test
04	insurance company adjustment	86588	direct streptococcus screen
05	adjustment, patient	87072	culture by commercial kit, nonurine...
12011	simple suture--face--local anes.	87076	bacterial culture, anaerobic, with GC...
29125	application of short arm splint; static	87086	urine culture and colony count
29425	application of short leg cast, walking	90703	tetanus injection
45378	colonoscopy--diagnostic	90782	injection with material, subcutaneous or
45380	colonoscopy--with biopsy	92516	facial nerve function studies
50390	aspiration of renal cyst by needle	93000	Electrocardiogram--ECG with interpret...
71010	chest x-ray, single view, frontal	93015	Treadmill stress test, with physician...
71020	chest x-ray, two views, frontal & lat...	96900	ultraviolet light treatment
71030	chest x-ray, complete, four views	99070	supplies and materials provided
73070	elbow x-ray, AP and lateral views	99201	OF--new patient, problem focused
73090	forearm x-ray, AP and lateral views	99202	OF--new patient, expanded
73100	wrist x-ray, AP and lateral views	99203	OF--new patient, detailed history and...
73510	hip x-ray, complete, two views	99204	OF--new patient, comprehensive history..
73600	ankle x-ray, AP and lateral views	99205	OF--new patient, comprehensive history..
80019	19 clinical chemistry tests	99211	OF--established patient, minimal
80061	lipid panel	99212	OF--established patient, problem focused
82270	blood screening, occult; feces	99213	OF--established patient, expanded
82947	glucose screening--quantitative	99214	OF--established patient, detailed...
82951	glucose tolerance test, three specimens	99215	OF--established patient, comprehensive..
83718	HDL cholesterol	99394	established patient, adolescent, per...
84478	triglycerides test	99396	established patient, 40-64 years, per...
85007	manual differential WBC		
85022	hemogram, automated, and manual...		

Payments _____

Remarks _____

Diagnosis 465.9

Index

4